Color Atlas and Text of

SPORTS MEDICINE
IN CHILDHOOD AND ADOLESCENCE

Edited by

Nicola Maffulli
MD MS PhD MIBiol FRCS(Orth)
Senior Registrar and Clinical Lecturer,
Department of Orthopaedic Surgery
University of Aberdeen Medical School
Aberdeen, UK

M Mosby-Wolfe

London Baltimore Dogotá Boston Buenos Aires Caracas Carlsbad, CA Chicago Madrid Mexico City Milan Naples, FL New York Philadelphia St. Louis Sydney Tokyo Toronto Wiesbaden

Copyright © 1995 Times Mirror International Publishers Limited

Published in 1995 by Mosby-Wolfe, an imprint of Times Mirror International Publishers Limited

Printed by Grafos S.A. Arte sobre papel, Barcelona, Spain

ISBN 0 7234 1700 8

For full details of all Times Mirror International Publishers Limited titles, please write to Times Mirror International Publishers Limited, Lynton House, 7–12 Tavistock Square, London WC1H 9LB, England.

A CIP catalogue record for this book is available from the British Library.

Library of Congress Cataloging-in-Publication Data applied for

Project Manager:	Linda Kull
Developmental Editor:	Claire Hooper
Cover Design:	Lara Last
Production:	Jane Tozer
Index:	Wendy Adamson
Publisher:	Geoff Greenwood

Contents

Preface

The number of youngsters in their early teens who practise regular exercise is increasing from year to year. Intensive training and high-level competition start at an ever decreasing age, and several medical bodies have issued guidelines on participation of children in competitive sports. Associated with the beneficial physiological, psychological and social aspects of exercise are the still largely unknown long-term effects of high-level sport.

The multifaceted aspects of modern Sports Medicine and the complexity of the issues involved make the subject exciting and challenging. Professionals dealing with young athletes must be conversant with the many aspects of a child's body to provide care and coach youngsters to their full potential. This illustrated guide outlines some of the effects of sports participation in young athletes. It should be remembered that only a few controlled studies have been performed, and that, inevitably, factual evidence is somewhat biased.

The informed, comprehensive and authoritative thoughts of leading researchers from Europe and North America on several hot topics in Sports Medicine in this age group are presented in the guide. As editor, I was in the hands of my authors, and at the mercy of the themes they wrote about. How very safe hands they proved to be!

I hope that the chapters presented add to the knowledge of those professionals already caring for young athletes, and stimulate them to do more, and better.

Nicola Maffulli
Aberdeen
Scotland, UK

Contributors

John Aldridge FRCS
Consultant Orthopaedic Surgeon, Coventry and
Warwickshire Hospital, Coventry, England, UK.

Neil Armstrong PhD FIBiol FPEA
Professor of Exercise Science,
Physical Education Association Research Centre,
University of Exeter, UK

Elena Ballarin
Centro di Studi Biomedici Applicati allo Sport,
University of Ferrara,
Ferrara, Italy

Chiara Borsetto
Centro di Studi Biomedici Applicati allo Sport,
University of Ferrara,
Ferrara, Italy

Francesco Conconi MD
Professor of Biochemistry,
Centro di Studi Biomedici Applicati allo Sport,
University of Ferrara,
Ferrara, Italy

Manolis Gavalas MB ChB FRCS
Senior Registrar in Accident and Emergency Medicine,
Whipps Cross Hospital, London, UK

Peter Helms PhD FRCP
Professor of Child Health,
University of Aberdeen,
Aberdeen, UK

David Jones PhD
Professor of Sports Science,
The School of Sport and Exercise Sciences,
University of Birmingham, UK

John King FRCS
Senior Lecturer and Consultant Orthopaedic Surgeon
Director, The Academic Department of Sports
Medicine,
The London Hospital Medical College, UK

C. Terence Lee MD
Resident in Obstetrics and Gynecology, University of
California, Irvine, Department of Obstetrics and
Gynecology, Orange, CA, USA.

Ze'ev Levita MA PhD
Consultant Psychologist,
Integrated Child Health Service, Greenwich,
London, UK

Nicola Maffulli MD MS PhD MIBiol FRCS(Orth)
Senior Registrar and Clinical Lecturer in Orthopaedics,
University of Aberdeen Medical School, Aberdeen,
Scotland, UK.

Lyle J. Micheli MD
Director, Division of Sports Medicine, Children's
Hospital, Boston, USA

M.E. Mills
Department of Physiology, University College London,
London, UK

Gabe Mirkin MD
Associate Clinical Professor,
Georgetown University, School of Medicine,
Maryland, USA

John Myers FRCS
Consultant in Accident and Emergency Medicine
Department of Accident and Emergency, Newham
General Hospital, London, UK

Pasquale Patrizio MD
Research Fellow, University of California, Irvine,
Department of Obstetrics and Gynecology, Orange, CA,
USA.

Craig Sharp BVMS, MRCVS, PhD, FIBiol
Professor of Sports Science, The University of Limerick,
Limerick, Ireland.

Paul M. Taylor DPM
Clinical Assistant Professor, Division of Orthopedics
(Podiatry), Georgetown University Hospital,
Washington, D.C., USA

George Thabit MD
Fellow in Sports Medicine, Children's Hospital, Boston,
USA

Joanne Welsman PhD
British Heart Foundation Research Fellow
Physical Education Association Research Centre,
University of Exeter, UK

1. Children in Sport: Questions and Controversies

Nicola Maffulli

Introduction

In Western societies, youngsters in their early teens may have already undergone intensive training and high level competition for several years in sports like gymnastics, swimming or tennis. This is probably due to the 'catch them young' philosophy, and to the belief that, to achieve international standing in later sporting life, intensive training should be started before puberty.

Increasing concern has led some medical bodies to issue guidelines regarding participation of children in competitive sports. Although the risks of high-level sport in these youngsters are currently unknown, an epidemic of sports injuries has been predicted as children change from free play to the stereotyped demands of the specialised patterns of movement imposed by a single sport.

In this chapter, some of the positive and negative effects of sports participation by young athletes will be revealed. Keep in mind that only a few controlled studies have been performed, and that, therefore, the evidence presented is inevitably biased.

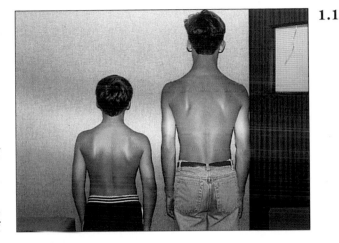

1.1

1.1 Familial shape or sports-induced paramorphism? These two brothers are both tennis players. Note the same degree of lowering of the right shoulder in both of them.

Physical, cardiovascular and muscular effects of sports participation

The physiological determinants of exercise performance mature during childhood and adolescence. Growth and development and also training produce marked increases in strength and endurance. The effects of physical training are thus difficult to separate from those of puberty.

Studies involving children have detected a wide range of results, from growth retardation to no effects at all. Although physical activity is required for normal growth, the minimum needed has not been identified, and the ill effects of intensive training have not been fully clarified.

In girls, research has focused on menarche and menstrual disorders. Several studies on the age of menarche, and the incidence and duration of menstrual disturbances in young athletes engaged in intensive training, have recently been carried out. With few exceptions, menarche appears to be delayed in athletes. Girls engaged in intensive training also show an increased frequency of menstrual irregularities. Factors that could influence the time of menarche, such as genetic influences or nutritional status, have not however been systematically controlled in these studies.

In boys, skeletal maturation was followed in athletes engaged in cycling, rowing and ice hockey from 12–15 years of age. Regular physical activity was found to have no quantifiable effects on the growth of young male athletes.

1.2

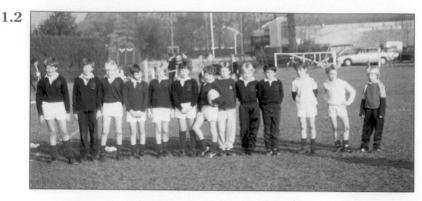

1.3

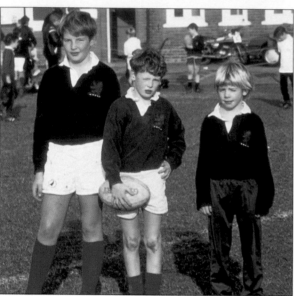

1.4

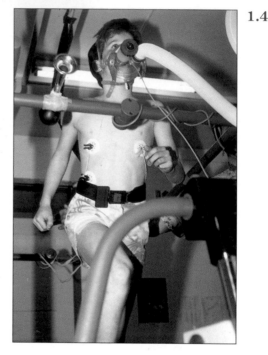

1.2, 1.3 The extreme variability in size in children of the same age (11 years) is shown. In this mini-rugby team, all the children are born within the same calendar year. There is a difference of 15 cm and 8 kg between the shorter and the tallest one. The child holding the ball is on the 50th centile for height and weight.

1.4 The high-tech environment of a modern sports physiology laboratory for the thorough assessment of the young athlete. The child is connected to gas analysers and electrocardiograph, and wears a safety belt to prevent injuries.

The response of a given athlete to a particular training regimen is due to inherited factors; only 30% approximately of the maximal oxygen uptake (VO_2 max.) and maximal force and power of top class competitors can be accounted for by training, although indices of submaximal exercise capacity are only partially genetically determined.

Young athletes undergoing vigorous training were found to be taller, to have less body fat and higher VO_2 max. than sedentary controls. For example, 34 boys aged 12–16 engaged in competitive middle- and long-distance running were compared with 56 controls not undergoing intensive training. The runners had been training for 2–5 years, and had less body fat and lower resting heart rates. Statistically significant differences were only achieved between the 16-year-olds. The young runners in this study also had larger heart volumes and a higher VO_2 max., relative to body weight and respiratory capacity.

1.5

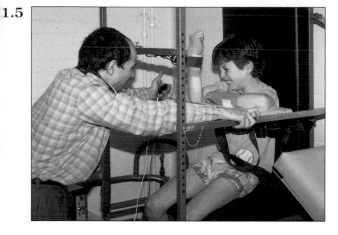

1.6

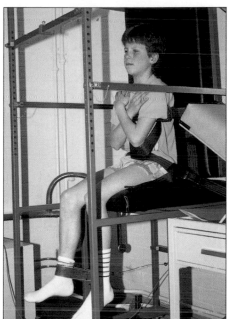

1.5, 1.6 A custom-made apparatus to test maximal isometric voluntary strength exerted by the elbow flexor and knee extensor muscles.

The histochemical and biochemical effects of endurance and sprint training were studied on the vastus lateralis muscles of 16- and 17-year-old boys. Endurance training resulted in a significant increase of type I and IIA fibre areas, together with increased activity of some of the enzymes of the Kreb's cycle. In the same study, sprint-trained boys showed a significant increase in the activity of glycolytic enzymes.

Few controlled studies have dealt with the trainability of muscular strength in children. Pre- and post-pubescent children of both sexes can significantly increase their muscular strength following resistance training. The traditional view is that the potential to develop strength is not at its maximum before puberty.

Nevertheless, pre-pubescent children could have a greater muscular strength trainability than an older age group, and increase significantly the muscular strength of both upper and lower limbs after appropriate resistance training. When interpreting the effects of a strength training programme, one should appreciate that the natural increase in strength in boys reaches its maximum approximately one year after the growth spurt, while in girls this occurs during the period of growth spurt itself.

Intensive training may result in staleness. There have been a number of reports detailing a fatigue syndrome in top class athletes. However, no controlled studies have been performed. Some possible important contributing factors to fatigue include an increased predisposition to viral infect-

ions, fatigue from overtraining or a combination of physical and psychological fatigue analogous to the 'burn out syndrome' reported in other contexts. Sports-mediated immune response alterations may play a major role in determining increased susceptibility to infections.

Sports injuries

Some studies have shown that 3–11% of school-aged children are injured each year due to sports activity. Physical characteristics can play a major role in the choice of a sport and also on the pattern of injuries. For example, marked joint laxity may result in a child's preference for gymnastics, but is associated with recurrent sprains and dislocations, and with low back pain.

During the growth spurt, adolescents are particularly vulnerable to injuries, partially at least due to the imbalance between strength and flexibility. The huge increase in participants and in the amount of training and competition has resulted in children incurring injuries that were previously seen almost exclusively in adults.

The skeletal system is extremely plastic in children, and shows pronounced adaptive changes to intensive sports training. The long-term effects on bone of participating in intensive training during the period of growth and development are still obscure. Low-intensity training can stimulate bone length, but high-intensity training may inhibit it.

1.7

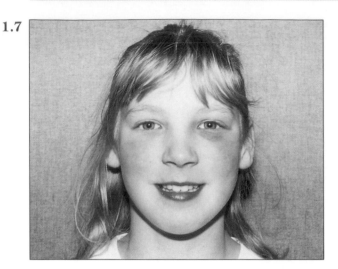

1.7 A fading haematoma of the left orbit is, fortunately, the only consequence of being hit by a tennis ball during a match.

1.8

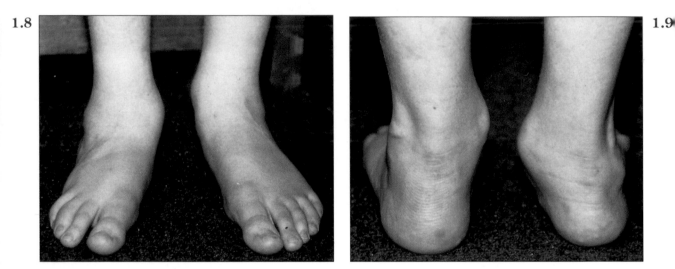

1.9

1.8, 1.9 To each his/her sport. This young athlete suffers from congenital hypoplasia of the leg, accompanied by a four-toe foot and marked valgus deformity of the hind foot. A weight-bearing sporting activity would cause serious problems due to the resulting severe biomechanical imbalance of the lower limb. The child is a successful swimmer.

1.10

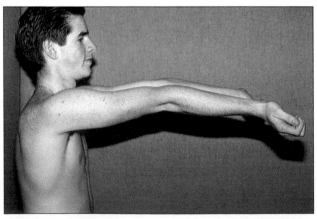

1.10 A predisposing factor to sports injuries. This degree of elbow hyperextension would be normal in a girl gymnast.

1.11

1.12

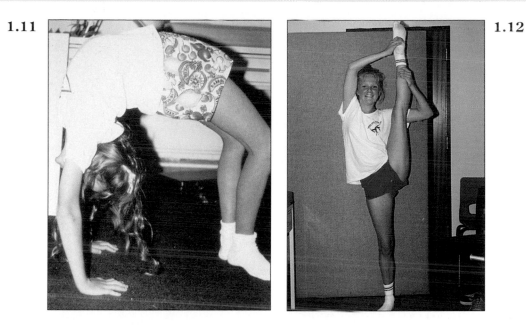

1.11, 1.12 These girls show the extreme flexibility achieved by modern successful artistic gymnasts.

1.13

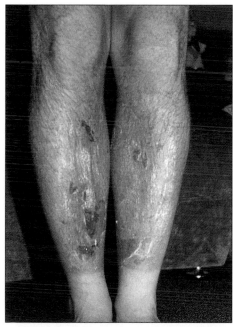

1.14

1.15

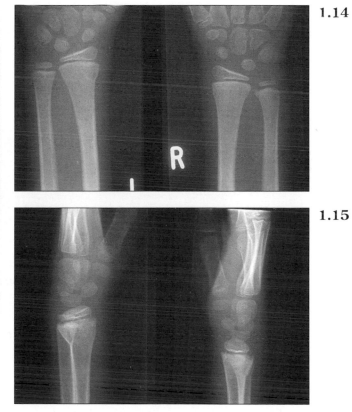

1.13 Not a sports injury, but equally serious. This tennis player, with extremely fair skin, has played for six hours in the south of Spain July sun, in a temperature of 38°C. Beyond risking dehydration, he has serious sunburn which needed hospital treatment.

1.14, 1.15 Bilateral greenstick radial fracture in a footballer: the result of a bad tackle. These undisplaced fractures heal without consequences in 3–4 weeks.

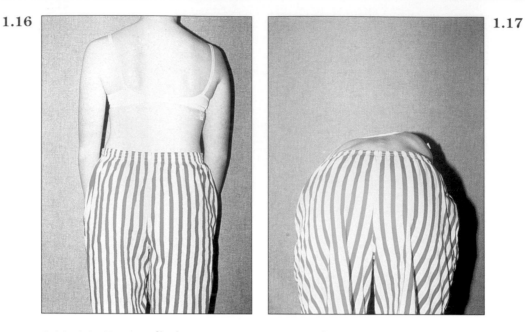

1.16, 1.17 True scoliosis in a young swimmer. There is lowering of the right shoulder, and, on forward flexion, a gibbus is seen.

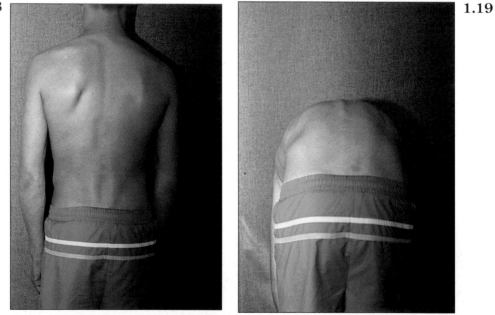

1.18, 1.19 'Tennis shoulder'. Compare with **1.16, 1.17**, and note absence of gibbus.

1.20 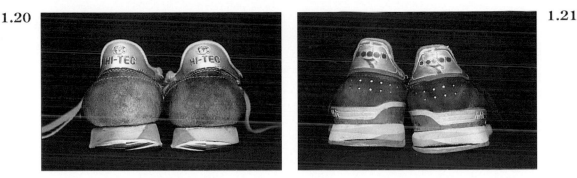 **1.21**

1.20, 1.21 It is not necessary to examine the feet of these young middle distance runners to know that one has hindfoot supination on the left, and the other marked hindfoot pronation on the right.

1.22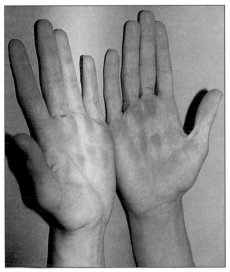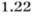

1.23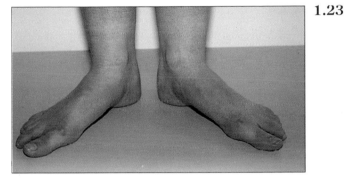

1.22, 1.23 The effects of repeated micro trauma on skin: extensive callosities of the hands and feet.

Sports injuries could impair the growth mechanisms, with subsequent damage for life. Physiological loading is beneficial, but excessive strains may result in serious injury to the weight-bearing joint surfaces. Due to the presence of growing cartilage, and the process of growth itself, the skeletal system of a young athlete is more prone to specific types of injuries. In addition, the ligaments of children are 2–5 times stronger than the cartilage and the bone of the epiphysial plate to which they are attached. This results in a greater likelihood of fracture of the epiphysial–metaphysial junction rather than the ligamentous tears seen in adults.

Overuse injuries are characterised by chronic inflammation due to repeated microtrauma. Young athletes may develop a group of overuse injuries termed 'osteochondroses'. Common sites are the posterior aspect of the calcaneus (Sever's disease), the tibial tubercle (Osgood–Schlatter disease), and the lower pole of the patella (Sinding–Larson–Johansson syndrome). The small carpal and tarsal bones may also be affected.

Young athletes are therefore at risk of developing stress lesions to these susceptible growth areas. In childhood, compression stress fractures may occur more commonly than the oblique type seen in adults. Endurance training regimens are probably responsible for at least 60% of all overuse injuries sustained. They could be avoided by appropriate changes in training programmes.

In the case of injury, probably the first therapeutic measure is rest. At high performance level, it is important to know whether an alteration of training regimen after an injury can maintain fitness and ensure rapid healing. Very little research has been performed in this area, although in one study that replaced endurance running with endurance cycling for four weeks, it was observed that maximal aerobic power and sub-maximal running performance for moderately trained women runners was maintained.

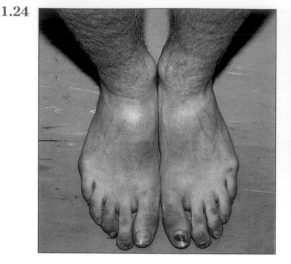

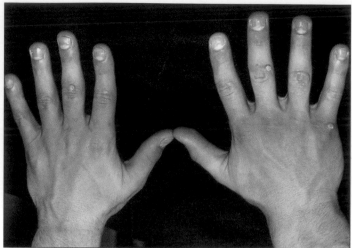

1.24 An overuse injury: subungual haematoma in a young middle distance runner.

1.25 The observance of basic hygiene rules is crucial: this young wrestler with verrucae infected three other members of his club.

Psychological effects

Young competitors suffer increased stress and anxiety due to competition. Parents may influence the outcome of a competition, potentially inducing a greater prevalence of aggression in the young athlete. This has led to the extreme position of calling for a complete ban of high-level competition for pre-adolescents because of the possible long-term deleterious effects. An outline of the psychological effects of intensive training on young athletes is part of another chapter in this atlas.

Conclusions

The physiological responses to training in children appear to be similar to those found in adults and, in the short term at least, seem beneficial. Definitive statements about the effects of intensive training on young athletes cannot yet be made. However, concerns about physical and psychological injury remain, and it is likely that the age of the child and the particular sport should influence the type and intensity of training.

Health professionals dealing with young athletes should be aware of these issues. Children are not just adults in miniature, and they should not be assumed to be capable of the same amount and quality of exertion as adults. Probably, it is safe to follow the 'ten per cent rule', which advocates progressing the intensity of any training programme no more than 10% a week.

Preparation and performance standards should take into account the chronological and biological age of the participants, and their physical and psychological immaturity. All adults dealing with high-standard athletic children should not exploit the youngsters, but maintain their state of health while helping them to improve their athletic performance.

A better insight into the different aspects of training is needed so that serious damage to children in high level competition is avoided. When planning a training programme, the physiological maturation process through which the children pass should be considered. Time is needed for a growing child to incorporate his own body changes, and probably little room is left at this critical stage for developing speed, strength and resistance.

However, recent evidence from the UK shows that intensively-trained young athletes do not appear to be at risk of serious injury. Whether this is due to the structure of the sport, or to a fierce selection process making the skeletal system more resistant to trauma, is still under study.

1.26

1.27

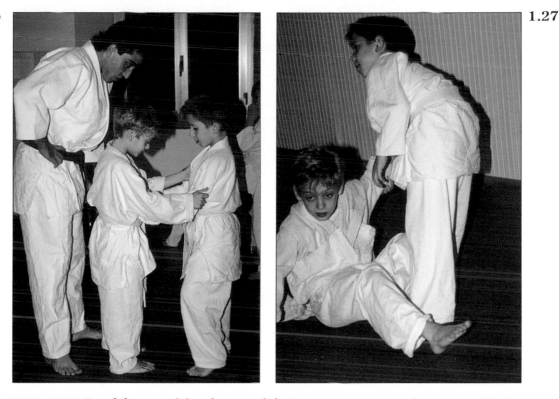

1.26, 1.27 Careful supervision by an adult is necessary to teach proper athletic movement, and to avoid accidents.

Suggested reading

Bonen, A. and Keiser, H.A. (1984) Athletic menstrual cycle irregularities: endocrine response to exercise and training. *Phys. Sportsmed.* **8**: 78–90.

Dalen, N. and Olson, K.E. (1974) Bone mineral content and physical activity. *Acta Orthop. Scand.* **45**: 170–174.

Ekblom, B. (1971) Physical training in normal boys in adolescence. *Acta Paediatr. Scand. Suppl.* **217**: 60–62.

Fagard, R., Bielen, W. and Amery, A. (1991) Heritability of anaerobic power and anaerobic energy generation during exercise. *J Appl. Physiol.* **70**: 357–362.

Keast, D., Cameron, K. and Morton, A.R. (1988) Exercise and the immune response. *Sports Med.* **5**: 248–267.

Larson, R.L. and McMahon, R.O. (1966) The epiphysis and the childhood athlete. *J. Am. Med. Ass.* **196**: 607–612.

Lysens, R., Steverlynck, A., van den Auweele, Y., Lefevre, J., Renson, L., Claessens, A. and Ostyn, M. (1984) The predictability of sports injuries. *Sports Med.* **1**: 6–10.

Maffulli, N. (1989) Skeletal system: a limiting factor to sports performance? A brief review. *J. Orthop. Rheumatol.* **2**: 123–132.

Maffulli, N. (1990) Intensive training in young athletes. The orthopaedic surgeon's view point. *Sports Med.* **9**: 229–243.

Maffulli, N. (1991) Injuries in young athletes: some epidemiological considerations. *Sports Med. Soft Tissue Trauma* **3**: 11–12.

Maffulli, N., Capasso, G. and Lancia, A. (1991) Anaerobic threshold and performance in middle and long distance running. *J. Sports Med. Phys. Fit.* **31**: 332–338.

Maffulli, N. and Helms, P. (1988) Controversies about intensive training in young athletes. *Arch. Dis. Child.* **63**: 1405–1407.

Maffulli, N. and Pintore, E. (1990) Intensive training in young athletes. *Br. J. Sports Med.* **24**: 237–239.

Maffulli, N., Testa, V., Lancia, A., Capasso, G. and Lombardi, S. (1991) Indices of sustained aerobic power in young middle distance runners. *Med. Sci. Sports Exer.* **23**: 1090–1096.

Malina, R. (1983) Menarche in athletes: a synthesis and hypothesis. *Ann. Hum. Biol.* **10**: 1–24.

Malina, R.M., Meleski, B.W. and Shoup, R.F. (1982) Anthroponetric, body composition, and maturity characteristics of selected school-age athletes. *Pediatr. Clin. North Am.* **29**: 1305–1323.

Micheli, L.J. (1983) Overuse injuries in children's sport: the growth factor. *Orthop. Clin. North Am.* **14**: 337–360.

Ogilvie, B. (1979) The child athlete: psychological implications of participation in sport. *Ann. Am. Acad. Sci.* **445**: 47–58.

Ramsay, J.A., Blimkie, C.J.R., Smith, R., Garner, S., MacDougall, J.D. and Sale, D.G. (1990) Strength training effects in prepubescent boys. *Med. Sci. Sports Exerc.* **22**: 605–614.

Rowland, T.W. (1990) Developmental aspects of physiological function relating to aerobic power in children. *Sports Med.* **10**: 255–266.

Rowley, S. and Maffulli, N. (1990) Gli effettti psicologici dell'allenamento intenso in giovani atleti. *Med. Sport* **43**: 49–53.

Wilkins, K.E. (1980) The uniqueness of the young athlete: musculoskeletal injuries. *Am. J. Sports Med.* **5**: 377–382.

2. Foot Injuries

Paul M. Taylor

Children's foot injuries in sports more often involve overuse rather than trauma. Overuse injuries are due to a low grade stress applied repeatedly to the same area over a period of time.[6] Examples of this may be simple blisters or calluses, or more serious injuries such as Achilles tendinitis. They usually develop gradually and, at least initially, do not limit activity. Acute injuries, such as sprains or fractures, will occur suddenly and usually require cessation of activity (**Table 2.1**).

Treatment will vary depending on the type of injury. An acute fracture, sprain or dislocation must be evaluated, X-rayed, possibly reduced and adequately immobilised as soon as possible.[7] Overuse injuries can initially be dealt with using the RICE concept: Rest, Ice, Compression and Elevation (**Table 2.2**). This initial treatment is directed at reducing the localised inflammation. However, it is also important to identify the cause of the overuse injury and take appropriate steps to stop the injurious events. If a child has chronic arch pain due to plantar fasciitis secondary to excessive pronation, this must be controlled with shoe modifications or orthotic devices before the symptoms can subside. Children, including young athletes, are prone to develop muscle imbalance, especially around the period of adolescent growth spurt, and appropriate stretching and strengthening programs are generally indicated.

In dealing with most foot injuries, a treatment concept of initial control of pain and inflammation, identifying the cause of the injury, and establishing a program to compensate for any structural or biomechanical imbalances will assure a quick recovery and prevent recurrence of the injury.

Injuries of skin and nails

Blisters

The repetitive motion between the foot and the sock creates significant shearing forces between the layers of the skin. As the heat, pressure and friction build up, the layers of skin may begin to separate and fill with fluid. This microscopic sequence of events results in a blister.[4] Initial treatment should include draining the fluid with a sterile needle, leaving the roof of the blister intact. A gauze dressing should be applied. Povidone cream helps to dry the lesion. Within a few days, the denuded area of skin under the blister should begin to heal and be less tender. If the skin becomes loose at this point it should be trimmed away.

Table 2.1.

	Overuse Injury	Acute Injury
History	No recollection of specific injury	Usually recalls time of injury
Onset	Gradual	Sudden
Pain	Mild–moderate	Moderate–severe
Mechanism of injury	Repetitive microtrauma	Acute trauma
Effect on activity	Modify or reduce activity	Stop activity

Table 2.2.

RICE

R est

I ce

C ompression

E levation

2.1

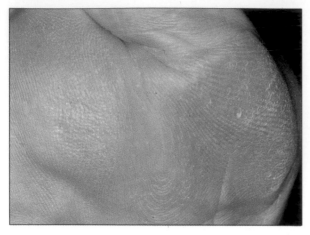

2.1 Callus formation is a normal thickening of the skin to protect areas of excessive pressure.

2.2

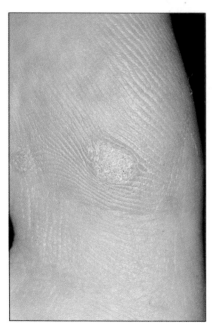

2.2 A plantar wart can be differentiated from a normal callus by the pulpy surface and the skin lines will go around the wart rather then continuing through the callus.

When children develop blisters, it is important to check that they have not outgrown their shoes. Wearing two pairs of socks or using socks designed to reduce shear will prevent blister formation. Applying vaseline, prior to participation, to an area that is prone to blister formation will also help.

Although most blisters heal uneventfully, the child and parents should be advised to observe the area until healed, as infection and cellulitis can be a complication.

Calluses

Callus formation is a normal protective mechanism of the body **(2.1)**. The epidermis will thicken in areas of excessive pressure to provide more protection. If an area of callus is asymptomatic, it should be left alone. Symptomatic callus can be self-treated with weekly reduction with a callus file or pumice stone, and daily application of hand cream or lotion. Children do not generally develop painful corns or calluses but, when they do, professional treatment should be obtained to debride the callus and evaluate for a shoe insert or padding. In children, an area commonly believed to be a painful callus could be a plantar wart.

Plantar warts (verruca)

Warts on the soles of the feet are commonly seen in adolescents. Blisters or abrasions on the feet and risks of exposure at pools or locker rooms increase the potential for exposure to the virus that causes these lesions. Initially, they may appear to be a callus, but warts show a more irregular surface. The skin lines continue through callus, but are interrupted by verrucas **(2.2, 2.3)**. A verruca will also be more painful, especially when applying pressure to the area.

2.3

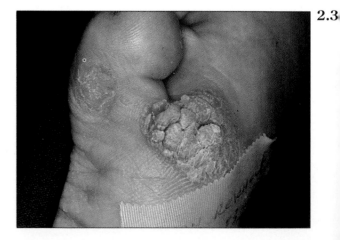

2.3 A plantar wart can become enlarged and painful.

Early treatment may consist of applying over-the-counter medications which consist primarily of mild concentrations of salicylic acid. These are applied daily and covered with a small bandage. Unfortunately, unless started very early, this strength of medication is not usually successful for the plantar verruca. Because of the pressure on the bottom of the foot, these lesions are pushed inward, indenting the surface of the skin. The wart itself does not penetrate the deeper layers of skin. Stronger acids such as 60% salicylic or monochlorocetic acid or blistering agents such as Cantherone(R) are successful when applied professionally. However, to the young athlete, the disadvantage with these is that the treatment may take several weeks and can be painful, interfering with their sporting activity.

Another option of treatment is curettage under a local anaesthetic or freezing with liquid nitrogen. This may require 5–7 days of inactivity after the surgery, but the overall treatment time is shorter.

Athlete's foot (tinea pedis)

Perspiration associated with physical activity and standing in common showers exposes the athlete to a high risk of fungal infections of the feet. In younger athletes, the acute type of tinea pedis with burning, itching and cracking between the toes is most common (**2.4**, **2.5**). However, the athlete who shows a reddish, dry, scaly change on the soles may also be infected with the more chronic type of tinea pedis.

Treatment of tinea pedis is usually successful with products currently available over the counter. Initial treatment should start with medications that contain undecylenic acid, tolnaftate, or clotrimazole. The topical anti-fungal agents should be continued for at least three weeks, even though the symptoms may improve in four or five days. Continuing the treatment will help prevent recurrence. In addition, the athlete should be advised to dry the feet well, change socks frequently and to apply an antifungal powder in the shoes on a daily basis. In resistant cases, the use of oral anti-fungal medication such as griseofulvin or ketoconazole may be necessary. In these cases, however, a positive KOH slide preparation or culture should be obtained first to confirm that the fungus is the aetiologic agent. For severe tinea pedis both the local treatment and oral medication may be needed for three or four weeks.

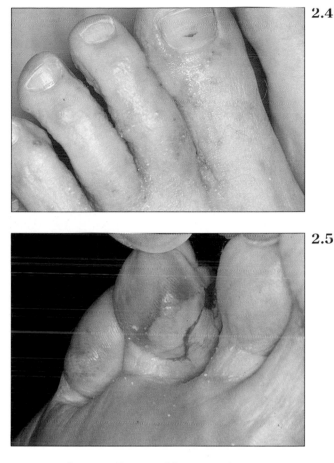

2.4

2.5

2.4, 2.5 Tinea pedis. In addition to the common cracking and itching between the toes, tinea pedis can progress to a more vesicular type eruption (**2.4**) or become inflamed and macerated (**2.5**). When changes such as this occur, a secondary yeast or bacterial infection should be suspected.

Ingrown toenails

Ingrown toenails can be an annoying problem to the young athlete. The condition may be caused by improperly trimming the nails, picking at the corners of the nails, or, in some cases, a hereditary tendency for the corners of the nails to curl inward. The mild cases show some irritation along the edge of the nail (**2.6**), while the more serious cases occur when the edge of the nail cuts into the skin and an infection develops (**2.7**).

2.6

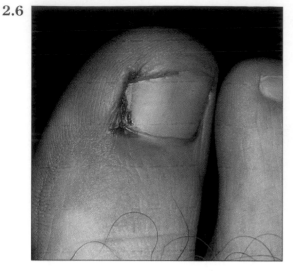

2.7

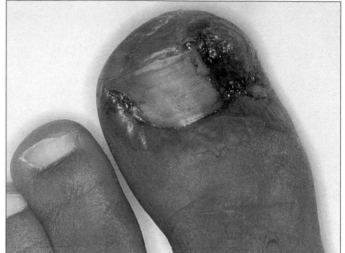

2.6 Ingrowing nail. At the early stages, an ingrown nail will show an inflammation of the nail fold, dry blood and pain on pressure.

2.7 A severe ingrown toenail will show swelling, drainage, malodour and the formation of granulation tissue around the nail.

Treatment for the mildly infected ingrown toenail includes soaking in warm Epsom salt solution (two teaspoons/quart of water) for 15 minutes, twice a day. This is followed by applying a topical antibiotic ointment to the corner of the nail, gently massaging the skin away from the edge of the nail. The more serious or recurring infected ingrown toenail may require surgical correction. Under a local anaesthetic, the offending portion of nail can be removed and then the soaks and antibiotic ointment applied. Another surgical option is to remove the side of the nail, including the nail matrix or root. This can be accomplished either by surgically resecting the nail matrix or by applying liquid phenol to destroy the matrix. Both techniques should provide a permanent correction.

Prevention involves teaching children proper techniques of cutting nails. They should be cut straight across, slightly rounding the edges so as not to leave a point. Children should be cautioned against picking the nails or pulling off the front edge. Sock and shoe sizes should be checked frequently to ensure that they have not been outgrown.

Black toenails

Black toenails are the result of bleeding under the nails. They may be either acute or chronic. The acute type of bleeding under the nail (subungual haematoma) occurs with a sudden forceful, trauma to the nail without lifting it off. This causes a bleeding which builds up under the nail and will turn black or blue (**2.8**). Due to the pressure which builds up under the nail, this type of injury can be very painful. If the blood does not escape spontaneously with loosening of the nail, then the haematoma should be drained as soon as possible. This can be done by using a lancet designed to puncture the nail, or drilling small holes in the nail plate. A paper clip can also be heated, while being held with pliers, and, by touching the nail plate, a hole in the nail will be produced, allowing escape of the blood. Two holes should be placed in the nail to allow adequate escape of blood. A sterile compression dressing should be applied to prevent additional bleeding under the nail. Follow-up care includes removing the bandage, warm Epsom salt soaks, then reapplying a bandage. This treatment, if carried out within 24 hours of the injury, will generally prevent loss of the toenail.

Chronic black toenails occur with an injury of repeated low-grade stress, such as tennis, where the foot slides forward in the shoe with only a slight amount of bruising under the nail. This is not very painful, but does cause discoloration of the nail. No treatment is needed in the absence of symptoms and the discoloured portion of the nail will slowly grow out. However, precautions should be taken to make sure shoes and socks fit properly to avoid repeated injury to the nails, as this may lead to damage of the nail root and permanent deformity of the nail (**2.9**).

2.8

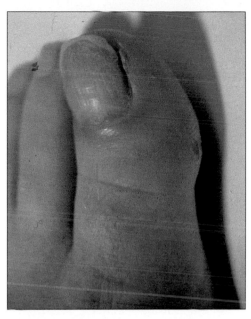

2.8 Acute sub-ungual haematoma.

2.9

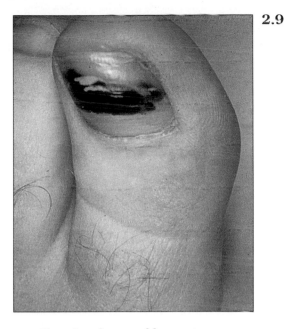

2.9 Chronic sub-ungual haematoma.

Foot and ankle sprains

Sprains are a common malady for the athlete. The ankle is most often affected, but the joints of the foot may also suffer similar injuries.[2] Sprains should be classified at the time of injury as mild, moderate or severe. This will help in establishing the treatment plan and prognosis for return to activity. A mild sprain involves stretching of ligaments without rupture. A moderate sprain includes partial rupture of ligaments, and a severe sprain indicates rupture of ligaments and possible avulsion fractures. In children, attention must also be directed to possible epiphyseal injuries.

All sprains should be treated initially with RICE (**Table 2.2**). For mild sprains, this will suffice as treatment and the athlete should be able to return to activity, with proper strapping, in 1–3 days. Moderate sprains require more aggressive treatment, including X-rays and partial immobilisation with strapping or a soft cast. Return to activity will require 10–14 days with a strengthening programme and strapping or an ankle brace. Severe sprains require a longer period of immobilisation with a cast or cast brace for 2–3 weeks, followed with another 2–3 weeks of strengthening exercises, before returning to activity with the use of bracing or taping.

Structural and functional foot problems

Flat feet (pes planus)

Flat feet is a common term which refers to low longitudinal arch to the foot on weightbearing (**2.10, 2.11**). Some children can function very well with a low arch foot. Treatment should be considered when symptoms appear, or secondary problems develop as a result of the flat feet. Children with symptomatic flat feet will not always complain specifically about pain in the arch. In fact, their complaints will more often be non-specific, such as tiring easily with activity, not being able to keep up with other children, or generalised soreness in the feet, legs, knees and even the lower back. Flat feet are a contributory factor to femoro-patellar pain in athletes.[3] In the older child with flat feet, early development of bunions and hammer toes may occur.

Treatment for symptomatic flat feet will vary depending on the severity. Over-the-counter types of arch supports are adequate for mild problems, but for moderate to severe pes planus, custom-made orthotic devices should be considered.

2.10

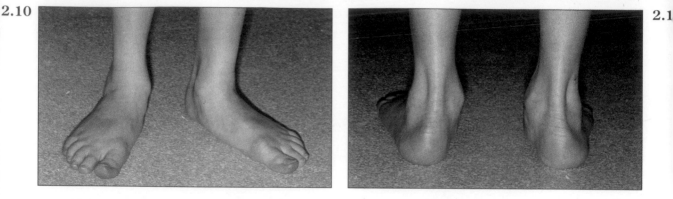

2.1

2.10, 2.11 Pes planus presents with a lowering of the arch, a forefoot abduction and an eversion of the calcaneus.

2.12

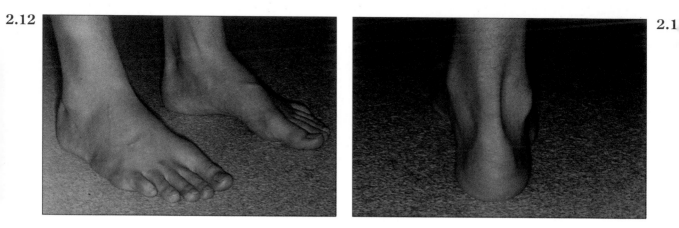

2.1

2.12, 2.13 Pes cavus presents with a high arch, forefoot adduction and a neutral or inverted calcaneus.

High arch feet (pes cavus)

The high-arch foot type is seen less commonly than the flat foot, but it may cause more problems and be more difficult to treat. The high arch foot is generally rigid, limiting the foot's ability to absorb shock. Children with this foot type will be prone to hammer toes, plantar fascitis, Achilles' tendinitis and stress fractures (**2.12, 2.13**).

Treatment should consist of stretching exercises, shoes with increased shock absorption, additional soft inlays in the shoes or custom-made soft orthotic devices.

Ankle equinus

Ankle equinus is a condition where the foot is plantar flexed at the ankle due to tightness in the gastrocnemius-soleus complex. Generally it is assumed that children are fairly flexible, but in the young athlete it is not uncommon to find a mild ankle equinus due to a tight calf muscle. Even in its milder form, this can have an adverse affect on the young athlete. For normal activity, there should be 10–15 degrees of dorsiflexion at the ankle (**2.14**). Without adequate dorsiflexion, the athlete will appear to be running on his toes. During the gait cycle, there will be an early heel lift. The changes in the normal biomechanics brought on by the ankle equinus will cause strain of the midfoot, plantar fascitis and Achilles' tendinitis. Treatment is directed to developing a stretching programme to increase the dorsiflexion of the ankle. Children with this problem must continue a regular stretching programme, otherwise the condition will recur.

'Growing pains'

Young active children commonly complain of leg pain or cramping at night. This is often defined as **'growing pains'.** However, these symptoms may be due to functional or structural imbalances within the feet or legs.

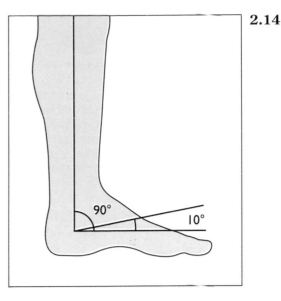

2.14

2.14 Normal ankle range of motion must allow at least 10 degrees of dorsiflexion during gait.

Conditions such as pes planus or pes cavus may be the cause of these pains. A child who complains repeatedly of this type of pain should be examined for foot problems and observed while walking. Any imbalance detected should be treated appropriately with stretching and strengthening programmes, shoe inserts or custom-made orthotic devices.

Haglund's deformity

Haglund's deformity is an enlargement of the posterosuperior border of the calcaneus. In the athlete, this can place increased pressure on the retro-calcaneal bursa or the Achilles' tendon. In young women, fashion shoes can cause irritation and swelling on the back of the heel due to the bone prominence (**2.15**).

Early treatment should include local ice to reduce the inflammation. Padding can be placed around the area to avoid shoe irritation. The irritation may be severe enough to warrant surgical excision of the bony prominence.

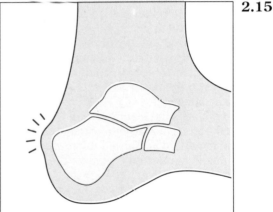

2.15

2.15 A Haglund's deformity is an enlargement of the posterior-superior border of the calcaneus which may cause pain and swelling on the back of the heel.

Juvenile bunions

A bunion deformity is an enlargement of the medial aspect of the head of the first metatarsal with a lateral deviation of the first toe. These usually develop as a result of an improper push-off during gait because of a foot imbalance, such as an excessively pronated or flat foot. Particularly in young women, these may become irritated earlier due to fashionable shoes and interfere with athletic activity.

The best treatment for bunions is early recognition and treatment. If caught early enough, and treated with orthotic devices to correct the foot imbalance and proper shoes, the progression of the bunion can be delayed or stopped.[5] If the bunions are not treated until they are in the later stages, then surgery may be needed. Unfortunately for the athlete, this may require an extended recovery period.

23

Toe deformities

Deformities of the smaller toes are not common in children. Mild congenital malformations resulting in slightly crooked toes may be seen occasionally, but these rarely are symptomatic, and do not require any treatment. If a child or parent reports progressive contraction of toes, this should be investigated. Any neurological problems should be ruled out as well as structural foot imbalances such as ankle equinus or pes cavus. When these structural problems are identified, they should be treated to avoid progression of the toe deformities, which can become painful if allowed to progress.

Overuse injuries

Tendinitis

The repeated motions associated with most sports frequently results in inflammation of the tendons around the foot and ankle. Achilles' tendinitis is frequently recognised but any of the tendons may be subject to overuse and inflammation. The anterior and posterior tibial tendons, peroneal tendons and even the flexor and extensor hallucis longus may be affected.

In the early stages the tendon sheath is primarily involved, and a tenosynovitis or a paratendinitis will result. If the condition is allowed to progress, or if there is an actual injury to the body of the tendon, a true tendinitis will evolve. Although not seen often in children, in the late stages a thickening and scarring of the tendon will lead to a tendinosis or possible calcific changes in the tendon. Eventually, a rupture of the tendon is possible. Because of the progressive changes in the tendon, any tendinitis should be treated early.

A tendinitis recognised should be treated with the usual RICE (Rest, Ice, Compression and Elevation) programme. Rest may only be a reduction in activity if symptoms are not severe. Ice should be applied after activity, and again at the end of the day. Compression can include the use of an elastic bandage or an elastic ankle brace. The foot should be kept elevated as much as possible. For a more severe tendinitis, oral anti-inflammatories may be used for 10–14 days. Cortisone injections for children or adolescents are almost never indicated.

A child prone to recurring tendinitis should be evaluated for structural imbalances which may be contributing to the problem.

Epiphyseal injuries

Epiphyseal closure generally occurs in boys between the ages of 14 and 16 and in girls between 12 and 14. Therefore, any child who complains of pain around a growth centre should be suspected of having an epiphyseal injury. This may only be an inflammation of the epiphysis related to overuse, or an epiphyseal fracture associated with acute trauma.

In the foot, the areas that may be affected include the calcaneal apophysis, the navicular bone, the heads of the metatarsals and the base of the fifth metatarsal.[1]

An epiphysitis should be treated aggressively with the general principles of RICE (**Table 2.2**). Rest should be enforced since repeated injury to the epiphysis can result in abnormal bone growth. If a fracture is suspected, then the foot should be immobilised.

Osteochondrosis

Osteochondrosis is a disorder in which the ossification centre of the bone undergoes aseptic necrosis, bony absorption and finally repair. This condition is seen most often at the femoral capital epiphysis and the tibial tubercle. The calcaneus, navicular and the heads of the metatarsals are most commonly affected in the foot although almost any bone can be involved (**Table 2.3**).

Table 2.3. Sites of osteochondrosis in the feet.*

Bone	
Talus	Diaz or Mouchet's disease
Cuneiforms	Buschke's disease
Navicular	Kohler's disease**
Calcaneal apophysis	Apophysitis, Sever's disease**
Fifth metatarsal base	Iselin's disease
Head of the metatarsals	Freiberg's disease**
Sesamoids	Trever's disease

*Tax, H.R. (1980) *Podopediatrics*, Williams and Wilkins, Baltimore/London.

**Kohler's, Sever's and Freiberg's disease are the most common - the others are rare.

Treatment includes protecting the involved area until the bone has healed, and avoiding damage to the surrounding cartilage. This will require cast immobilisation in most cases. On return to activity, the foot should be protected with additional shoe padding or orthotic devices.

Plantar fascitis/Arch strain

The plantar fascia is a thick, fibrous band which attaches on the inferior aspect of the heel and extends into the toes (**2.16**). The fascia aids in supporting the arch and prevents elongation of the foot, and may be overstretched in sports, resulting in plantar fascitis.

Treatment should be started with RICE (**Table 2.2**). The best method to allow the fascia to heal is the application of a low Dye or rest strapping. The strapping should be left on all the time, since even normal walking without protection will re-injure the fascia. If an athlete has problems with recurring plantar fascitis, then an orthotic device should be fabricated.

Metatarsalgia

Metatarsalgia is a vague term indicating pain in the area of the metatarsals. An attempt should be made to determine a more specific diagnosis. The pain may be due to a stress fracture, bursitis, neuroma or an osteochondrosis of the metatarsal head.

Initial treatment can be started with RICE (**Table 2.2**) and inserting a metatarsal pad in to the shoe. If the symptoms are not relieved within a few days, a more accurate diagnosis is needed in order to establish the most effective treatment regimen.

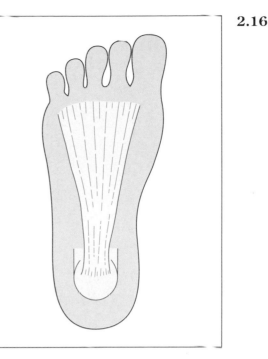

2.16

2.16 The plantar fascia is a thick, fibrous band which inserts across the plantar aspect of the calcaneus and sends multiple branches into the toes.

References

1. Ganzhorn, R. and Toy, B.J. (1990) Fractures to the fifth metatarsal. *Phys. Sportsmed.* **18(12)**: 67–70.
2. Irvin, W.O. (1992) Feet under force: treating sprains and strains. *Phys. Sportsmed.* **20(9)**: 137–144.
3. Newell, S.G. and Bramwell, S.T. (1984) Overuse injuries to the knee in runners. *Phys. Sportsmed.* **12(3)**: 80–92.
4. Ramsey, M.L. (1992) Managing friction blisters of the feet. *Phys. Sportsmed.* **20(1)**: 116–124.
5. Root, M.L., Orien, W.P. and Weed, J.H. (1977) *Normal and Abnormal Function of the Foot*, p.425. Clinical Biomechanics Corporation, Los Angeles, CA.
6. Taylor, P.M. and Taylor, D.K. (1988) *Conquering Athletic Injuries*, Leisure Press, Champaign, IL.
7. Tursz, A. and Crost, M. (1986) Sports-related injuries in children. *Am. J. Sports Med.* **14(4)**: 294–299.

3. Upper Limb Injury in Children's Sport

M. John Aldridge and Nicola Maffulli

Children are by definition growing and their developing skeleton is most vulnerable to injury. As in adults, soft tissue injuries do occur, but the most significant problems are related to the bone. Therefore, this chapter will deal mainly with skeletal injuries. It is important to have a basic overview of skeletal growth and development before talking about specific injuries.

The skeleton develops first as a scaffold of cartilage which is converted into bone by the process of endochondral ossification. The primary centres of ossification are situated in the diaphysis of long bones. Secondary centres develop at the proximal and distal ends, in the articular epiphyses. Further centres are the traction epiphyses at the insertion of major tendons. Articular epiphyses grow radially by division of cartilage cells around the epiphysis itself. Longitudinal growth occurs in the epiphyseal growth plate situated at either end of the long bones, between the articular epiphysis and the diaphysis.

Endochondral ossification is a very orderly process: cartilage cells divide and arrange themselves in columns to produce an organic matrix which calcifies into bone. Repetitive microtrauma may interfere with this process.

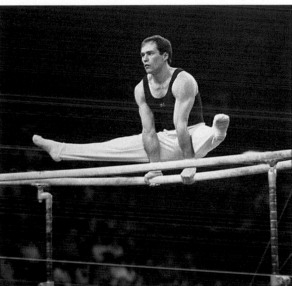

3.1 Compressive and rotational stresses. In gymnastics, compressive and rotational stresses are imposed on the wrist and elbow joints.

Acute injuries

Generalities

Children's fractures differ from those of adults because of the physical characteristics of their growing bone. Firstly, children's bone is more resilient and elastic, accommodating greater bending or rotational stresses before breaking.

When a child's bone does break, it may produce:

- The typical greenstick fracture of childhood. This is an angulated, incomplete fracture which tears the periosteum and cortex of the convex side while the cortex and periosteum on the concave side remain intact.
- The buckle fracture. This lesion occurs when compression forces are transmitted through the long axis of the bone. This is the adult equivalent of a compression fracture.
- Epiphyseal injuries. These are a group of fractures with no counterpart in adult life, occurring in the region of the epiphyseal growth plates. Shearing and avulsion forces are generally responsible for these injuries, but compression may play a significant role. The injuries are of special concern as the damage to the cartilaginous cells of the epiphysis may interfere with bone growth, causing subsequent deformity.

Salter and Harris classified injuries to the epiphyseal area into five Types. In Types I and II, the epiphyseal plate is intact. In this case, the prognosis

3.2

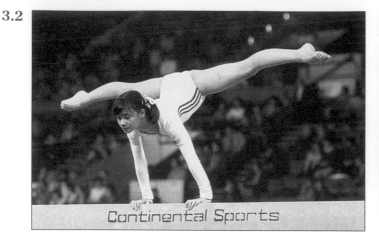

3.3

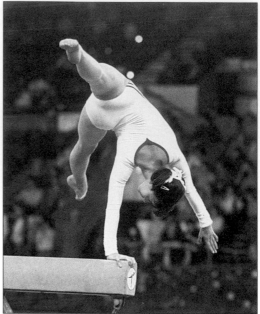

3.2, 3.3 Highly acrobatic manoeuvres in gymnastics may result in the upper limbs becoming weight bearing. At times, the whole body weight is sustained by one arm only.

3.4

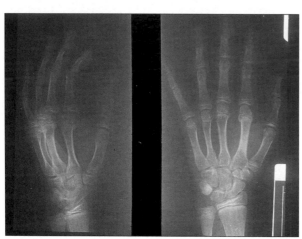

3.4 The result of an enthusiastic karate punch: a fracture of the neck of the second metacarpal.

is excellent and, after appropriate manipulation, growth continues undisturbed. In Types III and IV, the fracture runs through the joint surface and through the epiphyseal plate. Accurate reduction, either closed or surgical, is mandatory, so that the epiphyseal plate is correctly aligned. Failure to do this may lead to premature closure of the epiphyseal plate and disturbance of growth. Type V injury is quite often difficult to detect radiologically at the time of injury. It is a compression injury of the growth plate, so that growth may cease, and

deformity or disturbance of growth can follow.

In addition to greenstick and buckle fractures, and to epiphyseal injuries, children may also sustain complete fractures as in adults.

Healing of fractures in children proceeds much more rapidly than in adults, and remodelling of bone is an essential part of the healing process. Fractures that unite initially with some deformity can completely remodel, and appear totally normal later in life. Angular deformities are more easily corrected than rotational ones.

Principles of treatment

Treatment of children's fractures can be divided into four groups:

- Fractures with little or no displacement simply need protection in a splint until union occurs.
- Complete fractures with displacement need manipulation and immobilisation. It is not always important to achieve anatomical alignment of the bone, but rotational deformities must be corrected.
- In greenstick fractures, the angular deformity should be corrected, and the correction held in plaster.
- Fractures which require open reduction and internal fixation are rare in children. Open reduction and internal fixation is indicated in epiphyseal injuries with irreducible displacement and in fractures where a joint surface is involved.

3.5

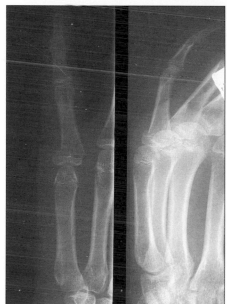

3.5 Hockey injury in a 13-year-old girl: a Salter Harris Type II injury of the basal phalanx of the little finger. Manipulation and strapping are standard treatment.

3.6

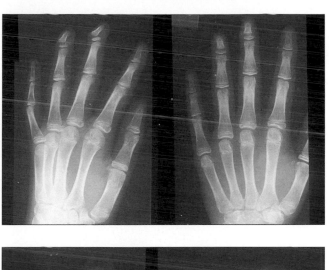

3.7

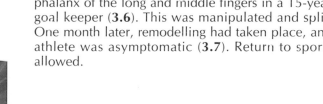

3.6, 3.7 A Salter–Harris Type I injury of the distal phalanx of the long and middle fingers in a 15-year-old goal keeper (**3.6**). This was manipulated and splinted. One month later, remodelling had taken place, and the athlete was asymptomatic (**3.7**). Return to sport was allowed.

3.8

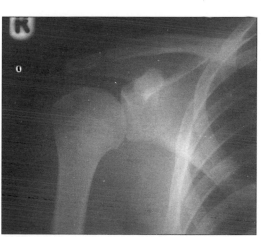

3.8 Fracture of the neck of the scapula due to a fall on the outstretched hand in a 14-year-old judo player. Conservative symptomatic treatment was instituted. The young athlete recovered full range motion of his shoulder in six weeks.

Specific upper limb injuries

Fractures of the clavicle

A very common injury in contact sports and in sports involving falls on the outstretched hand. A fall on to the shoulder itself can also produce this injury. The prognosis is excellent. Reduction is not necessary, and the child simply needs a sling to immobilise the arm until union occurs, generally in 2–3 weeks.

3.9

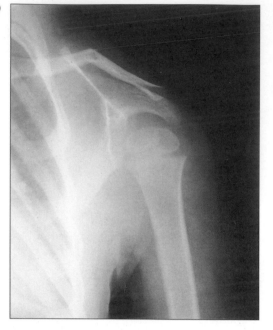

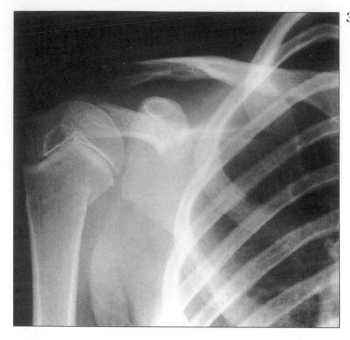

3.)

3.9 A fall from a horse. Landing on the shoulder resulted in a fracture of the clavicle in this girl.

3.10 Minimally displaced fracture of the neck of the humerus in a mini-rugby player.

Fractures of the humerus

Fractures of the upper end

These can be of two varieties. One is a fracture through the upper humeral epiphysis, usually the Salter Type II injury. The other is a fracture through the metaphysis which is seen particularly in older children. It can present as a buckled fracture or a complete fracture.

The displacement of a complete humeral fracture is often extensive, but it is rarely necessary to correct the deformity, as these fractures unite satisfactorily, and good remodelling takes place.

Fractures of the shaft of the humerus

The mechanism of injury is usually indirect. Typically, a fall on the arm causes a rotational injury to the upper limb. Conservative treatment with a hanging cast is sufficient.

Dislocation of the shoulder

This is rare in young children, and occurs in teenage life. The injury can be caused by a fall on to the outstretched hand or shoulder, although this mechanism is more likely to cause a fracture at the upper end of the humerus than a dislocation in this age group. When a dislocation does occur in older childhood or adolescence, reduction is necessary and immobilisation for three weeks in a sling is required. The risk of developing a recurrent dislocation of the shoulder is very high in this age group.

Elbow injuries

Elbow injuries during sport in childhood are common. These injuries cause much anxiety for several reasons:

- It is often difficult to interpret the radiographs of the elbow in growing children, which can make diagnosis quite difficult
- Damage to major vessels or nerves may occur.
- A number of children require operative reduction.
- The elbow is very liable to post-traumatic stiffness.
- Damage to the growth plate can cause subsequent deformity.

Supracondylar fractures

These occur in the lower part of the humerus just above the elbow joint. They can often involve the

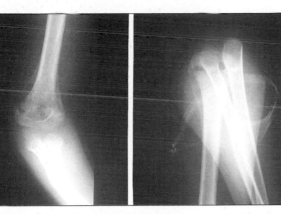

11

3.12

13

3.14

15

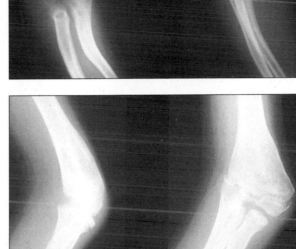

3.11–3.15 Evolution of a fracture of the distal humerus in a footballer. The fracture, which occurred when the chid was six years old (**3.11**), was manipulated, a slightly residual rotational deformity was accepted, and the patient was immobilised in a sling. Although remodelling took place at the age of 14 years (**3.15**), a bony deformity was evident. No surgery was carried out because the patient had accepted the deformity and the limitation in motion.

growth plate. The distal part of the humerus can displace posteriorly (more commonly) or anteriorly. These fractures should be manipulated and held either in flexion or in extension, depending on the type of fracture, in a splint. It is imperative to make sure that there is no associated brachial artery injury. It is often difficult to be certain that rotation is corrected, it is essential that this is achieved.

Early complications can lead to brachial artery damage and local nerve damage. Late complications can lead to:

- Ischaemic contracture: if blood supply to the forearm muscles has been interrupted, they become fibrous and shortened, causing flexion deformities of the fingers.
- Mal-union: if the fracture is not reduced correctly, deformity may persist. If this is unacceptable to the patient and his/her parents, the deformity must be corrected surgically.
- Post-traumatic myositis ossificans is common around the elbow joint. The traumatised soft tissues calcify causing stiffness and permanent limitation of movement. These fractures do not require physiotherapy treatment in this age group, and children should be allowed to regain movement slowly and gently.

3.16

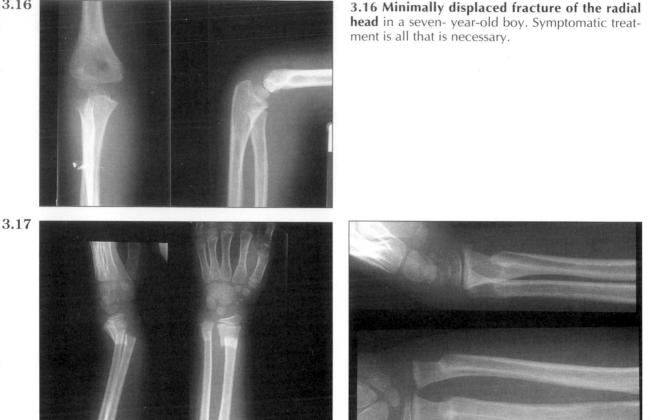

3.16 Minimally displaced fracture of the radial head in a seven- year-old boy. Symptomatic treatment is all that is necessary.

3.17

3.

3.17, 3.18 Complete fracture of the distal end of the radius and ulna in a seven-year-old boy. Despite incomplete alignment of the bone ends, after five months remarkable bone remodelling had taken place, and nearly perfect alignment had been restored (**3.18**).

3.19

3.20

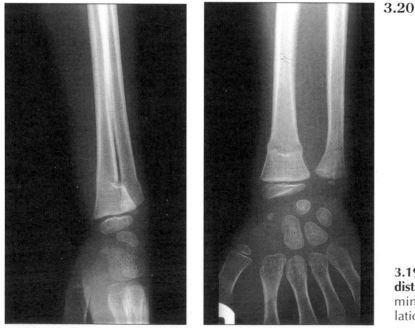

3.19, 3.20 Greenstick fracture of the distal end of the radius and ulna with minimal displacement. No manipulation is necessary in these cases.

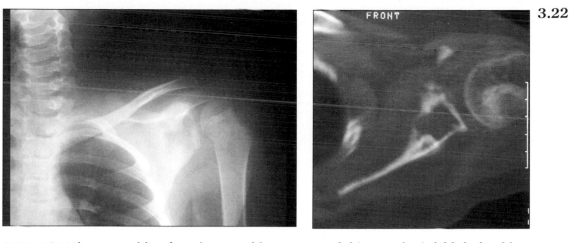

3.21, 3.22 Nine-year-old male swimmer with a two-month history of painful left shoulder. His GP had diagnosed impingement syndrome. Two months of treatment with modified rest, physiotherapy, ice packs and ultrasound were of no benefit. The left shoulder was slightly tender over the lateral end of the spine of the scapula. Motion was limited to 100° in abduction and about 120° in flexion. Radiographs showed a multilocular osteolytic area extending laterally from the scapular neck to the glenoid cavity (**3.21**). A CT scan in the horizontal plane showed erosion of the anterior and posterior cortex of the scapula (**3.22**). The tumour was resected 1cm medially to its medial margin through a posterior approach. No evidence of soft tissue involvement was found. Histology showed a giant cell tumour. Mobilisation was started the day after the operation. The child was subsequently treated by the oncologists. Six months after surgery, the patient was well. Movement was limited to about 90° in abduction and 110° in flexion. The shoulder was stable, despite post-operative retroversion of the pseudo-joint and the inevitable ligamentous damage. He has not been able to resume competitive swimming, but is leading an otherwise normal life three years after the operation. *Not all pains and aches in young athletes are due to injuries.*

Dislocation of the elbow

A relatively common injury in childhood, it can be complicated by fractures to the medial side of the distal humerus or fractures of the neck of the radius. The ulnar nerve may be damaged by the displaced elbow. Extreme caution should be exercised in rehabilitating these injuries, and premature return to sporting activities should be discouraged. The child should have regained a full range of movement before resuming sport.

Fractures of the forearm and wrist

Fractures of the radius and ulna

They are common injuries, generally due to indirect trauma from a fall on the outstretched hand. All levels of the forearm can be affected, although most fractures occur over the distal third. They generally present in one of three forms:

- A buckle fracture.
- A greenstick fracture, due to a combination of both vertical and rotational forces.
- Complete fractures due to considerable violence, such as falling from a horse or a bicycle.

These injuries are generally treated by manipulation and simple immobilisation in plaster.

Distal radial growth epiphysis injuries

Another common injury, the fracture is usually a Salter Type II, and reduction and immobilisation is generally sufficient.

3.23 **3.24** **3.25**

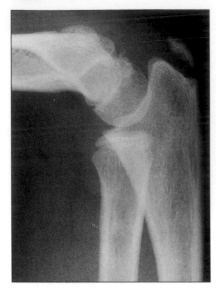

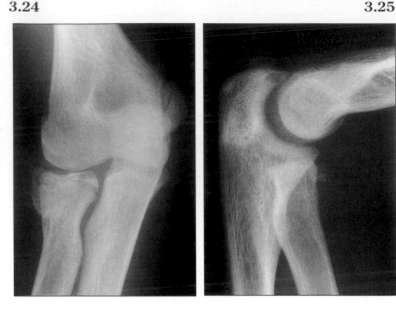

3.23 Fragmentation of the ole-cranic epiphysis in a gymnast. This represents an overuse injury of a non-articular epiphysis. Treatment is by rest.

3.24, 3.25 Articular osteochondrosis of the radial head (3.24). This is a well recognised entity in gymnasts, and results in progressive pain and limitation of motion. Eventually, excision of the radial head had to be performed (**3.25**). The young athlete never returned to gymnastics.

Overuse injuries

The normal process of skeletal development can be affected by repetitive stresses and, as a result, the normal growth process can become affected. The developing skeleton is particularly vulnerable during periods of increased growth such as the adolescent growth spurt. During this period, the epiphyses are very active and therefore vulnerable to stress. Also, body shape is changing rapidly, and adaptations have to be made in terms of the child's activities. Skeletal development is genetically determined and this influences how much stress can be placed upon the developing skeleton. The amount of stress that one child can sustain may be totally different to another. Therefore, one child may be able to play two or three games of football per weekend without developing an overuse problem, whereas another can only play one, and then suffer from an overuse injury.

Overuse injuries can cause breakdown in the normal process of endochondral ossification. When this happens, the descriptive term 'osteochondrosis' is used. Osteochondroses can be classified into:

• Non-articular osteochondroses, when a traction epiphysis is affected.

• Articular osteochondroses, when the articular epiphysis is involved.

• Epiphyseal plate osteochondroses, when the linear growth plate is damaged.

Articular and epiphyseal plates fail under compressive forces, whilst non-articular areas fail in tension. Upper-limb osteochondroses are much less common than those affecting the lower limb.

Non-articular osteochondroses

In the arm, the commonest affected area is where the triceps muscle inserts into the olecranon epiphysis. The condition presents with local pain and tenderness around the insertion of the triceps tendon. The child will complain of pain when supporting his/her body weight with the arms.

A radiograph may show fragmentation of the epiphysis, as one may see in other osteochondroses, but they are difficult to interpret because of normal variants in this region. It is not a common condition, but occurs most frequently in gymnasts. Treatment consists of a period of rest from upper limb activities. Symptoms usually settle over three months, and long-term problems are rare.

26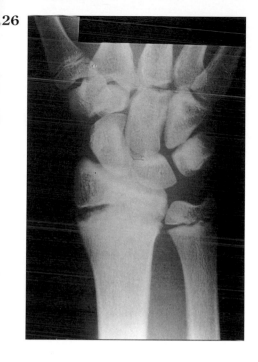

3.27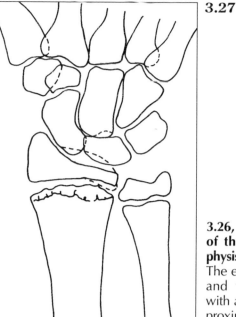

3.26, 3.27 Overuse injury of the distal radial epiphysis in a gymnast (**3.26**). The epiphysis is widened and slightly scalloped, with a ragged appearance proximally (**3.27**).

Articular osteochondroses

These are less common than non-articular ones, but are perhaps more important because of their long-term effects. They are of two types: one affects the whole epiphysis, the other only part of it. The latter condition is known as osteochondritis dissecans.

Osteochondritis dissecans

The knee is the most common site of this condition, but it can occur in any joint. It seems to be related to jarring activities, although constitutional factors are important. There appears to be a familial basis, as it frequently occurs in siblings. It is related to damage to the blood supply at a vulnerable time of epiphyseal development.

The elbow joint has been extensively studied in tennis and baseball, but gymnasts as well are at risk of the lesion. It generally affects the humeral capitellum, although the radial head can be involved.

OSTEOCHONDRITIS DISSECANS OF THE HUMERAL CAPITELLUM

The role of trauma in the production of this lesion has been well documented, although it can occur in non-sporting children. It occurs in the dominant arm in little league baseball pitchers. It is related to valgus loading of the elbow during pitching, so that the lateral side of the joint is repeatedly compressed. It has also been reported in boxers and divers.

In gymnasts, compression and rotation during weight bearing through the arm affect the elbow. Loading of the lateral side of the joint is increased by the physiological valgus of the elbow. These children present with elbow pain and some swelling. They often cannot fully extend the elbow, which is slightly tender over the lateral aspect. In general, initial signs and symptoms are minimal. The diagnosis is made on radiographs, but early diagnosis may require magnetic resonance imaging or computer tomography. The damaged area of the articular epiphysis can break away to form an intra-articular loose body.

If the condition is recognised early, conservative treatment is prescribed. Weight bearing on the upper limbs or stressing of the elbow are proscribed until healing occurs. When loose bodies are produced, they should be removed surgically. The long-term prognosis is worrying because the articular surface is damaged and the joint is not congruous. Early osteoarthrosis can therefore ensue.

OSTEOCHONDRITIS DISSECANS OF THE RADIAL HEAD

Osteochondritis dissecans of the radial head is a rare condition. It presents in a similar manner to that of the capitellum with local pain, swelling and limitation of joint motion. Again, diagnosis is by radiography. The treatment is along the lines of osteochondritis dissecans affecting the humeral capitellum.

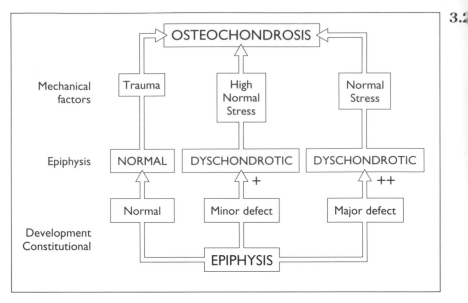

3.28 A schematic model for the production of osteochondrosis.

Osteochondrosis affecting a whole epiphysis

Occasionally, the whole epiphysis can be affected. Usually, the capitellum is involved, and the condition is known as Panner's disease. The blood supply of the whole area is impaired, and not simply of a segment of it, as occurs in osteochondritis dissecans.

The symptoms are pain, swelling and limitation of movement of the elbow. Diagnosis is radiological. The prognosis of the condition is not good. The lesion will heal, but the way of healing is important. If it results in a deformity, there will be incongruity of the joint, and an early osteoarthrosis could ensue.

Epiphyseal growth plate osteochondrosis

At times, due to repeated microtraumas, the epiphyseal growth plates fail. This is a relatively rare condition and only a few reports have been published. Fractures through the olecranon epiphysis have been reported in adolescent baseball players. The condition certainly occurs in gymnasts. It presents as pain in the posterior aspect of the elbow with local tenderness over the olecranon epiphysis. Elbow extension is decreased. Radiographs show widening of the epiphyseal line.

Following a period of conservative treatment, healing usually takes place. On occasions, the epiphyseal plate fails to fuse and surgery can be necessary to achieve this.

Stress-induced changes in the distal radial epiphysis are well recognised in gymnasts, and seem to be a sport-specific condition, although there is a case report of a skate-boarder with a similar problem. These children present with wrist pain associated with some swelling and local pain on weight bearing and rotational activities.

Radiographs show widening of the growth plate with failure of the zone of calcification. Treatment consists of rest to allow the epiphysis to recover. The prognosis is good, although growth can be interrupted, and the child may end up with a slight shortening of the radius compared with the ulna. This is an unusual and rare complication, and can be treated surgically. However, no long-term studies are available, and there is some evidence that these children may have to give up their sport.

Suggested reading

Chan, D., Aldridge, M.J., Maffulli, N. and Davies, A.M. (1991) Chronic stress injuries of the elbow in young gymnasts. *Br. J. Radiol.* **64**: 1113–1118.

Maffulli, N. (1990) Intensive training in young athletes. The orthopaedic surgeon's viewpoint. *Sports Med.* **9**: 229–243.

Maffulli, N., Chan, D. and Aldridge, M.J. (1992) Overuse injuries of the olecranon in young gymnasts. *J. Bone and Joint Surg. (Br. Vol.)* **74**-B: 305–308.

Maffulli, N., Chan, D. and Aldridge M.J. (1992) Derangement of the articular surfaces of the elbow in young gymnasts. *J. Pediatr. Orthop.* **12**: 344–350.

4. Lower Limb Injuries in Adolescence and Childhood

John King

Children are, for the main part, subject to all the problems of the athletic adult but carry additional disadvantages. They are more active and less wise; their skeleton is changing shape and size, and they have the relatively weak epiphyseal plate near the ends of the bones.

They have certain advantages. They usually carry less weight and have more elastic bones, so that the soft tissues are not subject to the same peaks of deformation as the adult. As a result, they have better shock absorbers.

Lesions of and around the hip joint

There are various sites around the hip that are weak as a consequence of open growth plates. Quite large pieces can be pulled off, particularly with sudden unexpected loads. The anterior inferior iliac spine (**4.1**) tends to rupture in football when the kicking foot is suddenly blocked, perhaps in a tackle, or more often when the foot hits the ground. It is pulled off by the reflected head of rectus femoris. In very similar circumstances, the psoas muscle can pull off the lesser trochanter (**4.2**).

The whole apophyseal plate of the ischium (**4.3**) can separate through the abnormal pull of the hamstrings; a good example is in cross-country running when the ditch being jumped is wider than first thought and the leading leg is overstretched.

More rarely, the anterior superior iliac spine can be pulled off (**4.4**) by the sartorius muscle in a bad gymnastic vault landing and the whole iliac crest apophysis can be pulled by the abdominal muscles, although displacement is most uncommon.

In all cases there is a good history of injury associated with severe, immediate, well-localised pain. X-rays usually confirm the diagnosis if awareness of the condition leads to a request for the appropriate views. Treatment is control of pain, rest and gradual resumption of activity as pain permits; this area is not amenable to the application of ice, as for the main part the avulsions are too

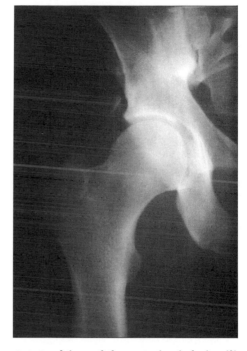

4.1 Avulsion of the anterior inferior iliac spine.

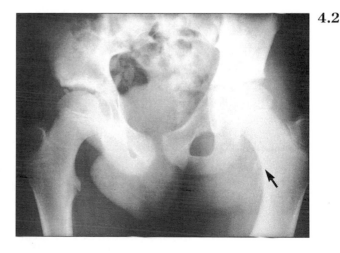

4.2 Avulsion of the lesser trochanter.

4.3

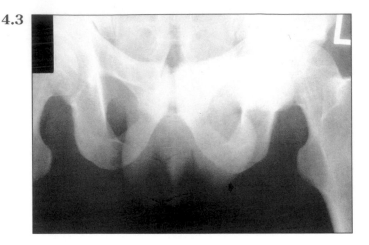

4.4

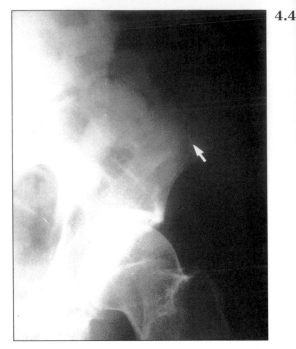

4.3 Avulsion of the ischium.

4.4 Avulsion of the anterior superior iliac spine.

deep. There is no indication for immediate surgery and late surgery is exceptional despite occasionally dramatic X-ray changes.

There may apparently be sports-related damage within the hip joint itself, but, as the aetiology of common hip conditions is not clear, it may be unfair to implicate sport in the causation. However, cessation of sport may be necessary in the management of the condition.

'Irritable hip' can occur at any age but is most common in children. It presents with a limp and the localisation of pain may be difficult. The child is usually brought along by worried parents and only examination reveals the painful restriction of motion of the hip joint. Full extension and/or abduction in flexion cause the pain. For the most part a precise cause is never found and the pain settles during a period of bed rest and observation. For this reason,the condition is often called 'observation hip'. X-rays and blood tests are usually normal and there is an argument that the children can be rested at home. In those cases where the radiological joint space is increased by 2 millimetres or more, there is a somewhat increased risk of Perthes disease (more accurately Legg–Calve–Perthes disease) occurring. Despite the benign evolution, X-rays and blood tests are mandatory to exclude the rare cases of tuberculosis or bone tumour that may present in this way.

Perthes disease affects the proximal femoral epiphysis usually in the age range 5–10 years. The aetiology is probably two or more episodes of raised intra-articular pressure leading to avascular necrosis of part of the head. The presentation is an 'irritable hip' with X-ray changes consisting of sclerosis of the femoral head (**4.5**). There are various grades of change reflecting the extent of the lesion and its probable outcome. The more complete the lesion the worse the outcome; the earlier its onset the better the outcome. Treatment varies between supervised neglect and surgery, the finer points of which are not appropriate to this volume.

Between the ages of 10 and 16, slipping of the upper femoral epiphysis is more common. It occurs mainly in boys and in two groups: the fat child with underdeveloped gonads (Frolich's syndrome) and the tall thin child undergoing a growth spurt. West Indian females seem more common in the second group but are still a substantial minority.

The child is frequently brought to medical attention after an injury in which the thigh has apparently become suddenly painful. Close questioning often reveals some premonitory discomfort; this is a common problem in that patients like an orderly life and often give their interpretation of cause and effect as the actual presentation of the problem (very common in bone tumours).

The pain is usually perceived in the knee because of the nerve supply from the hip (Hilton's Law) and there are very few cases in which there is not an X-ray of a normal knee in the envelope. The physical signs are of loss of internal rotation or even fixed external rotation and shortening of the leg. The external rotation of the foot in stance is by far

4.5

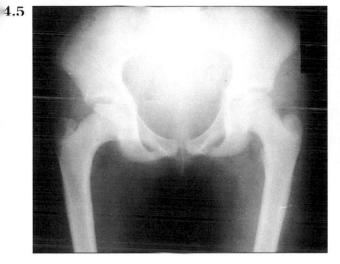

4.5 Perthes disease showing increased density and collapse of right femoral head.

4.6

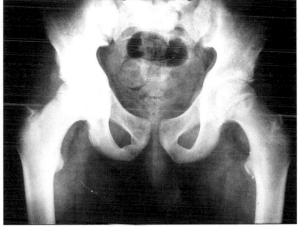

4.6 Anterior view of slipped upper femoral epiphysis. The changes are subtle but a line projected up the lateral side of the neck does not go into the head.

4.7

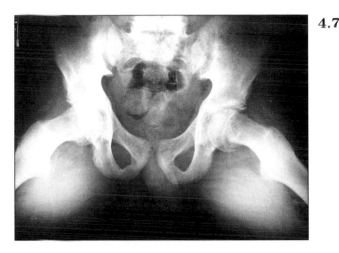

4.7 The lateral view of 4.6 shows clearly the umbrella-shaped epiphysis dropped backwards off its stem.

the most obvious sign and, with the child on the couch, internal rotation will be restricted or even impossible. Such physical signs demand an X-ray of the hip in both anteroposterior and lateral (**4.6, 4.7**) projections. The deformity is much easier to see in the lateral but there are well described criteria for its recognition in the anteroposterior radiograph. Treatment is surgical to prevent further displacement. It has been suggested that minor degrees of slip give rise to the loss of internal rotation, often seen later in life with 'pistol grip hips'.

Thigh injuries are non-specific to childhood except for the fact that the periosteum is more loosely attached and subperiosteal haematoma may occur. The story of an injury (see comments above) followed by increasing pain, particularly with sleep disturbance must alert the physician to a bone tumour or infection. Osteosarcoma (**4.8**) and osteoid osteoma (**4.9**) are the most likely and will have characteristic X-ray changes. Benign tumours such as simple bone cysts (**4.10, 4.11**) are most likely to present with a fracture (**4.12**) through the weakened area and are treated as a fracture; many of them will heal spontaneously after injury (**4.13**). Brodie's abcess or primary chronic osteomylitis is often best demonstrated with tomograms (**4.14**) and requires drainage (**4.15**).

4.8

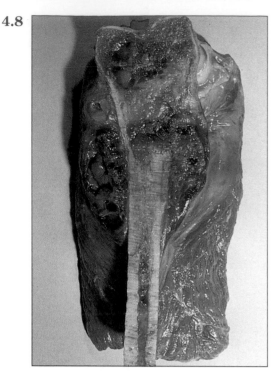

4.8 Osteosarcoma seen here in the tibia with bursting of the cortex and extension into the soft tissue.

4.9

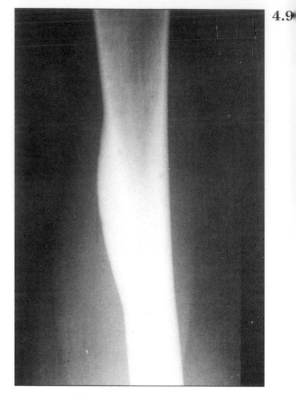

4.9 Osteoid osteoma with dense sclerosis asymmetrically placed in the mid part of the femur.

4.10

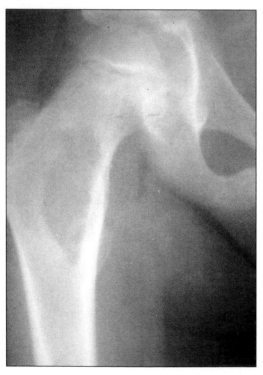

4.10 Unicameral bone cyst in the neck of the femur.

4.1

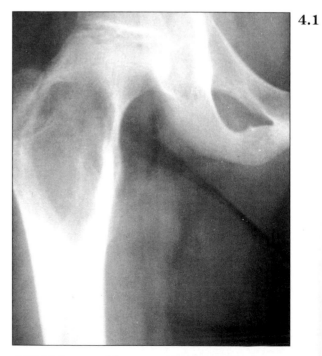

4.11 Unicameral bone cyst increased in size.

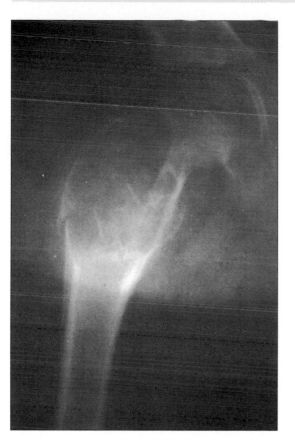

4.12 Unicameral bone cyst recently fractured.

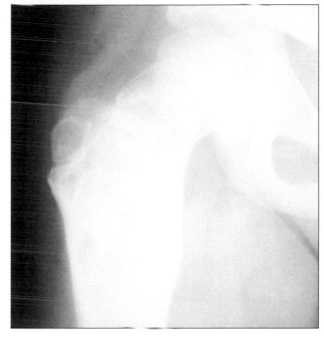

4.13 Unicameral bone cyst healed after the fracture.

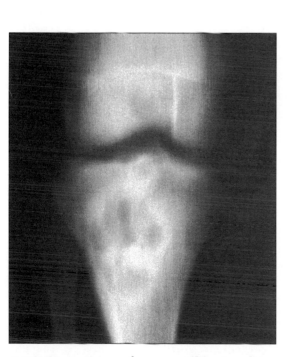

4.14 Tomogram of upper tibia to show Brodie's abscess.

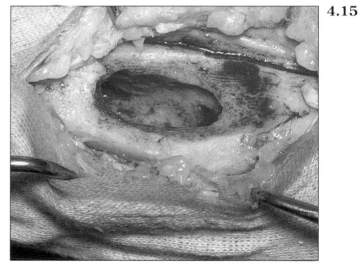

4.15 Operative photograph with drainage of Brodie's abscess.

4.16

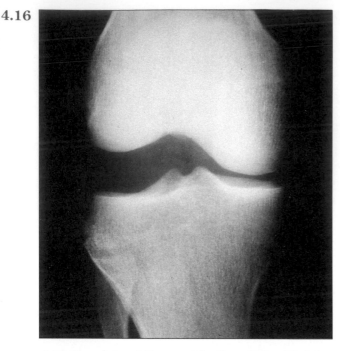

4.

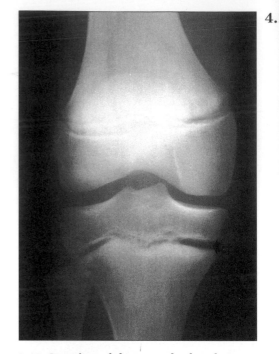

4.16 Torn lateral ligament in the adult with joint space opening.

4.17 Opening of the growth plate but not the joint in a child.

4.18

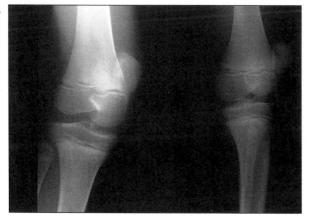

4.1

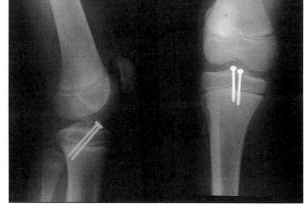

4.18 Avulsion of the anterior tibial spine by the anterior cruciate ligament.

4.19 Screw fixation of the fragment shown in 4.18.

Lesions of and around the knee joint

Injuries of the distal thigh merge with those of the knee. In the mature skeleton, valgus/varus stress tears the collateral ligaments (**4.16**); in the child, the epiphyseal plate is weaker than the ligaments and gives way (**4.17**). The knee may appear unstable and plain radiographs normal; a high index of suspicion is necessary along with stress X-rays, under anaesthesia if the pain is great. Treatment is immobilisation for four weeks.

Similar disproportion of strength produces the classical anterior cruciate lesion of childhood. The ligament stays intact but a large piece of the proximal tibia is avulsed (**4.18**). The history of injury is a flexion twisting, or hyperextension injury with immediate pain and swelling. X-rays are diagnostic and the fragment of bone can be screwed back (**4.19**).

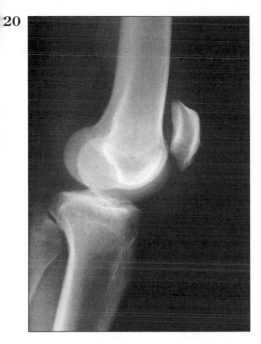

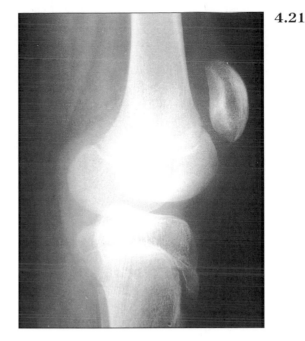

4.20 High patella not engaged in the femoral condyles.

4.21 Subluxed patella.

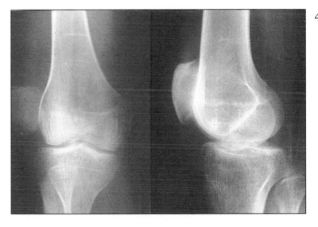

4.22 Dislocated patella.

The patello-femoral joint is often vulnerable, especially if the patella is a bit high and thus does not fully engage the femoral groove (**4.20**). Twisting of the leg with the knee slightly flexed may cause subluxation (**4.21**) or dislocation (**4.22**) of the patella. If it remains dislocated, the diagnosis is easy but spontaneous relocation can cause difficulties. The knee is swollen and the medial patellar margin is tender where the soft tissues have torn. Skyline X-rays are needed to exclude the marginal fractures (**4.23**) which, if untreated, can lead to loose bodies. As a basic rule in children, giving way on twisting is always patellar until proved otherwise. Meniscal problems in this group are very rare and almost always associated with a discoid meniscus with a history of painless clonking before the tear.

The extensor apparatus above the patella is rarely injured in children. The 'sleeve' injury of the patella occurs when the periosteal sleeve of the patella is stripped downwards in continuity with the tendon. The diagnosis is usually missed until the bone grows again in the empty pouch, producing the double patella appearance (**4.24**). Then it is too late to operate.

Traumatic cysts can occur in the patella ligament (**4.25**) in children, especially in divers who kneel on the edge of the pool as they climb out. These cysts have proved resistant to surgery (**4.26**) by comparison with similar lesions in older patients.

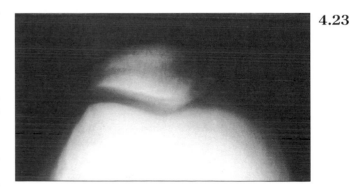

4.23 Marginal fracture of the patella.

4.24

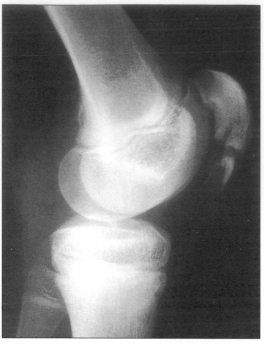

4.25

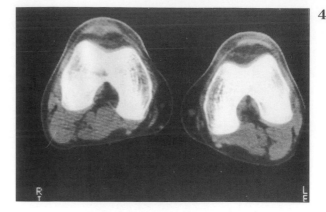

4.25 Computerised tomographic scan of a cyst in the patellar ligament.

4.24 'Double' patella. In this case, a rather small lower segment. This is *not* a fracture.

4.26

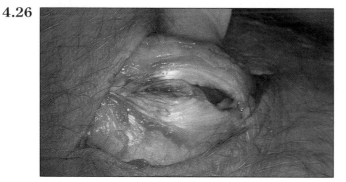

4.26 Operative photograph of a cyst in the ligament.

4.2

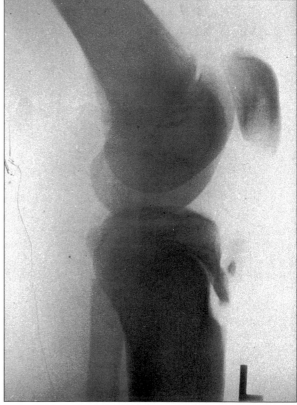

Perhaps the commonest lesion of the extensor apparatus is Osgood–Schlatters disease in which the tip of the elongated proximal epiphysis is elevated (**4.27**) by repetitive stress resulting in a painful lump (**4.28**) and radiological fragmentation and elevation. Treatment is restriction of activity to acceptable pain levels and protection of the bone lump from daily trauma by a neoprene sleeve. Only very rarely does the fragmentation give rise to symptoms in later life. At the other end of the tendon, at its patellar insertion, there may be pain associated with a small area of calcification which may respond to a carefully sited injection.

4.27 Elevated tibial tuberosity.

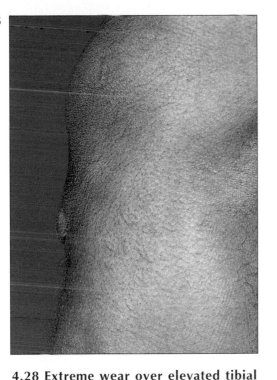

4.28 Extreme wear over elevated tibial tuberosity.

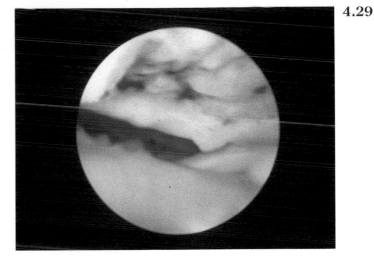

4.29 Arthroscopic appearance of a chondral separation.

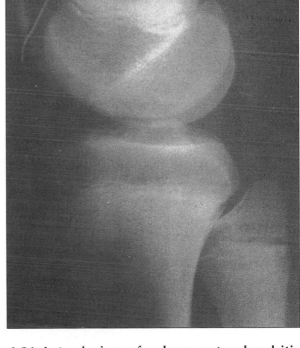

4.30 A chondral fragment removed from the knee.

Within the knee, osteochondral fractures may affect the weight-bearing articular surface of the femur as a consequence of a twisting injury. They present with a haemarthrosis; the X-ray may be helpful but the diagnosis may only be clear on arthroscopy (**4.29**). The fragment must be fixed back as it can represent a major part of the weight-bearing articular surface (**4.30**). This is not osteochondritis dissecans (**4.31**) which is an atraumatic lesion of the subchondral bone which can, nevertheless, separate (**4.32**); nor is it a growth anomaly (**4.33**).

4.31 Lateral view of a loose osteochondritis dissecans fragment. Note the drain.

4.32

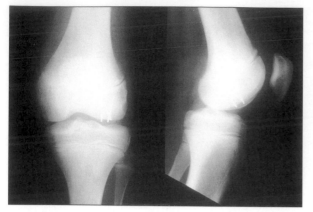

4.3

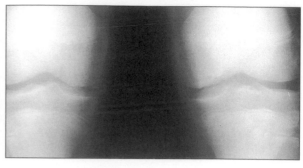

4.33 This is a growth abnormality and *not* osteochondritis dissecans.

4.32 Osteochondritis dissecans pinned using old fashioned nails. We would now use biodegradable pins.

4.34

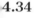

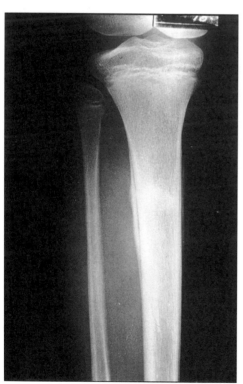

4.3

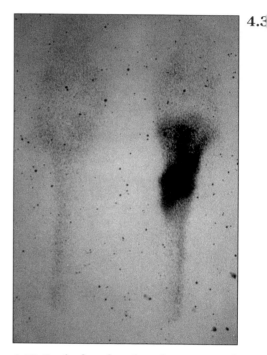

4.35 Typical technetium bone scan of an active stress fracture.

4.34 Late stress fracture of the tibia with extensive periosteal new bone.

The tibia (and more rarely the femur) may be the site of stress fractures (**4.34**). These occur as a consequence of repetitive load and inadequate recovery time so that fatigue failure takes place. The symptoms are of crescendo pain, the pain coming on sooner and sooner after the commencement of activity. Initial X-rays are normal but the fracture often becomes clear in later views. A Technetium diphosphonate bone scan is diagnostic (**4.35**). They must be distinguished from the tibial stress reaction which is a more physiological response to heavy use (**4.36, 4.37**). Treatment is reduction of activity to a pain-free level with a very gradual increase thereafter.

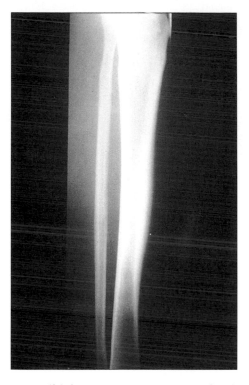

4.36 Tibial stress response to overload.

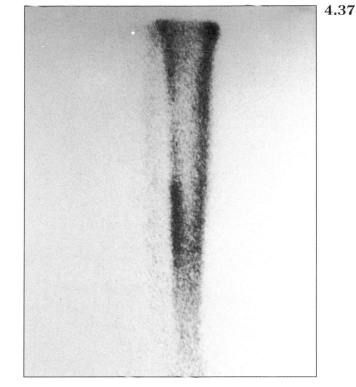

4.37 Technetium scan of tibial stress overload.
Compare this with the stress fracture shown in **4.35**.

Lesions of and around the ankle

The twisting injuries that cause the fractures in adults produce a different pattern of injury in the immature skeleton. Adduction force instead of breaking the fibula pulls open the distal fibular epiphysis. This almost always closes up and the only way to make the diagnosis is to find the well-localised tenderness at the site of the epiphysis (**4.38**). Treatment is immobilisation for two or three weeks until the pain subsides. Inversion injury causing the talus to spin pulling off a piece of bone (**4.39**) from the anterolateral corner of the epiphysis: the Tillaux fracture (**4.40**). Replacement of the bone fragment is necessary. Of more complexity is the triplane fracture that initially looks like a Salter type II injury (**4.41**). It is very difficult to reduce and may need open reduction and internal fixation.

Within the ankle, osteochondral fractures can occur. They are much smaller than in the knee and may be difficult to diagnose; a scan usually confirms them.

Apart from the obvious fractures which can occur at any time, the foot is the site of stress lesions rather more commonly than is realised. The classic

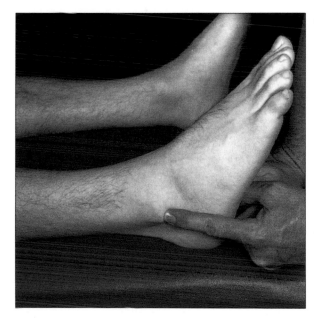

4.38 The site of tenderness in epiphyseal disruption.

4.39

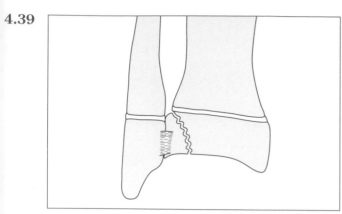

4.39 Illustration of Tillaux fracture.

4.40

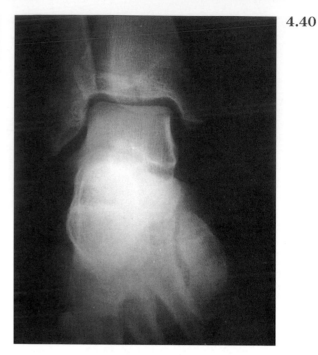

4.40 X-ray of Tillaux fracture.

4.41

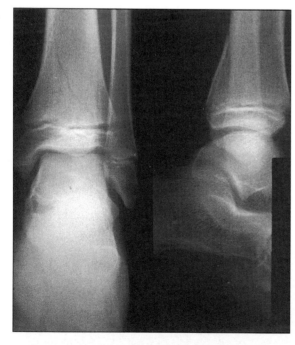

4.41 A Salter II fracture in which the epiphysis is slightly slipped and a triangle of bone from the metaphysis has come with it.

4.42

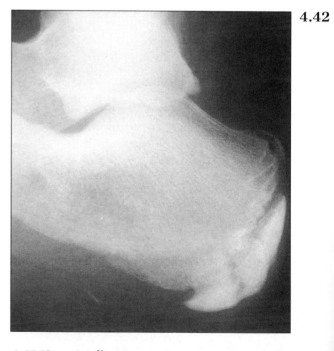

4.42 'Sever's' disease.

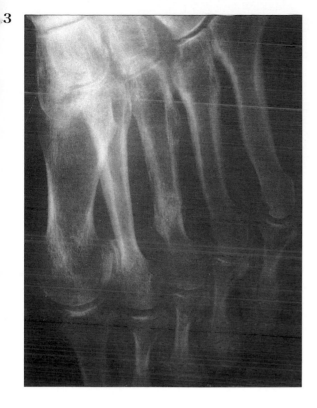

4.43 A stress fracture of the middle metatarsal.

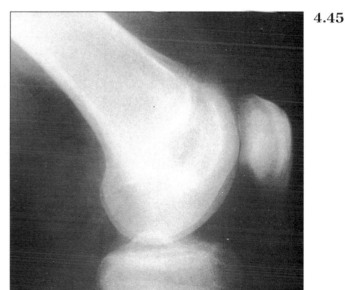

4.44 AP view of congenital bipartite patella. Note the gap and the superolateral position of the small fragment.

compression stress fracture of the adult calcaneum is rare but there may be pain and radiological fragmentation (**4.42**) of the calcaneal apophysis. This has been called Sever's disease. It presents with well-localised activity-related pain on the point of the heel. Devas in *Stress Fractures* (1975, Churchill Livingstone) takes these to be stress fractures but there is often a similar asymptomatic X-ray of the other side. The pain responds to rest and a shock absorber under the heel. The navicular is quite a common site of stress fracture and this is difficult if not impossible to see on an X-ray. The patient is often a young fast bowler, the pain is well localised and the treatment is rest. Occasionally it needs fixation. The stress fractures of the metatarsals are common, the history is diagnostic and the callus will show on the late radiographs (**4.43**).

Accessory bones may be a problem both in diagnosis and treatment. There are two particular sites. The bipartite patella shows on X-ray as a separate piece of bone on the superolateral corner of the patella (**4.44, 4.45**). The gap between it and the main part of the bone may be palpable. It is usually bilateral. It does not usually give rise to spontaneous pain but if the patella has been

4.45 Lateral view of bipartite patella.

4.46

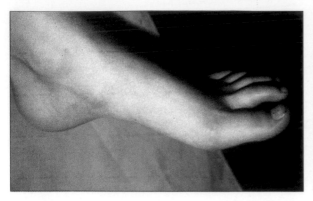

4.46 Typical bump of an accessory navicular.

4.47

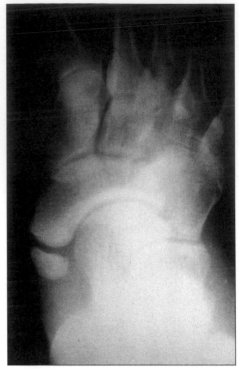

damaged, usually by a blow on the front, the symptoms of that may not settle until the segment is removed. The same problem occurs in the accessory navicular (**4.46, 4.47**) which is usually symptom free. If there has been a traction lesion, usually from eversion injury, the pain may persist until excision of the extra bone.

Suggested reading

4.47 X-ray of an accessory navicular.

Maffulli, N. (1990) Intensive training in young athletes. The orthopaedic surgeon's viewpoint. *Sports Med.* **9**: 229–243.

Maffulli, N., King, J.B. and Helms, P. (1994) Training in elite young athletes (the training of young athletes (TOYA) study): injuries, flexibility and isometric strength. *Br. J. Sports Med.* **28**: 123–136.

5. The Exercise Physiology of Children
N.C. Craig Sharp

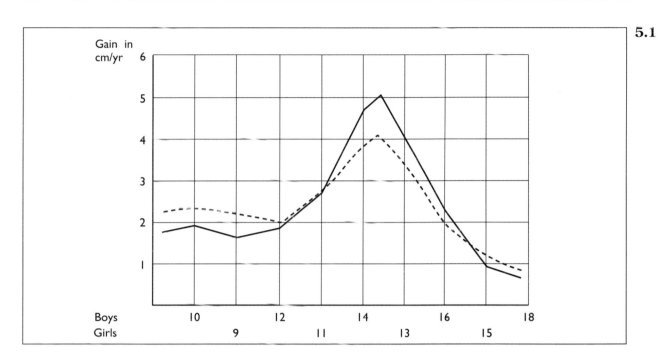

5.1 Graph of sitting height changes in children.

Size and weight

Children do not grow at an even rate. The marked increases of the adolescent growth spurt may lead to height changes of up to 15cm (6in) over the main two years of the spurt (**5.1**). As this occurs some two years earlier in girls, there is an age, around 11 to 12, when many girls will be bigger, heavier and stronger than their male peers. In the 1981 Melbourne marathon, the 11- and 12-year-old categories were won by girls.[25]

Playground and classroom bullying of boys by girls is then not uncommon. Also, physical development does not necessarily parallel chronology, which has implications for age-group sport. Many early-maturing athletes become discouraged when their slower-growing peers catch up, and some late-maturers may give up the unequal struggle and drop out of sport altogether.

Intense pre-pubescent training in girls, as in gymnasts, swimmers, runners and dancers, may delay puberty. For example, competition swimmers who only began the sport seriously after menarche, had a mean age of its onset of 12.5 years, while those who started very young entered menarche at 15.[11]

Scaling body-size data

A major problem in comparing some physiological parameters in young and older children, and in children with adults, concerns 'scaling' or normalising data for different body sizes[39] (**5.2**). Until recently, the use of ratio standards, e.g. ml $O_2.kg^{-1}$ body weight, was considered as adequate normalisation, although over 40 years ago Tanner[34] indicated that correlating body mass and physiological values could give misleading results. The fallacy involves a special case of the spurious correlation between indices. Thus young children (and small adults) appear to have unduly high maximum oxygen uptakes (if expressed as $ml.kg^{-1}$) and heavy adults appear relatively low. For example, a British rowing gold medallist at

51

5.2

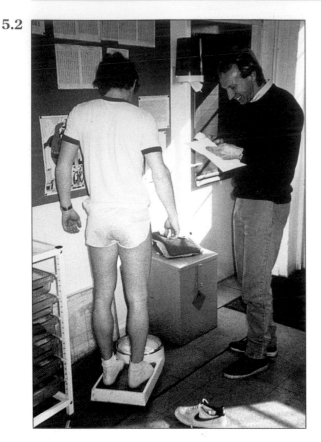

5.2 Weighing the subject: adequate normalisation?

Barcelona, with a body weight of 100kg, had a $\dot{V}O_2$(max) of 'only' 74ml.kg^{-1}.min^{-1}.

Thus, some authors[21] propose that the physiological values be divided by body mass recorded in the units kg$^{-2/3}$ as power function ratio standards. Whereas these proposals do not fall within the brief of this book, they are a pointer to the future.

Estimation of body fat

Using skinfold callipers for estimating body fat in children (**5.3, 5.4**), is relatively unreliable although it is still useful to compare the same child at different ages. At eight years of age, girls have approximately 18% body fat, and boys 16%, but during the growth spurt the fat in girls tends to increase to about 24–26% at 17, with the percentage in boys tending to diminish to 12–15% in later teenage years.

5.3

5.4

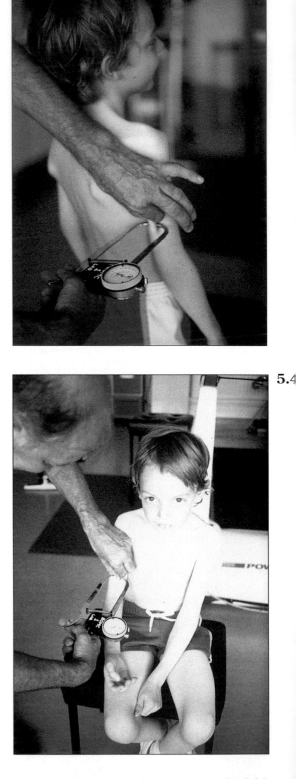

5.3, 5.4 Estimation of body fat by skinfold callipers.

5.5

5.6

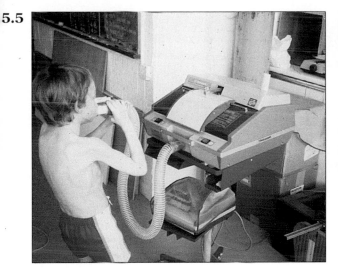

5.5 Respiratory parameter assessment.

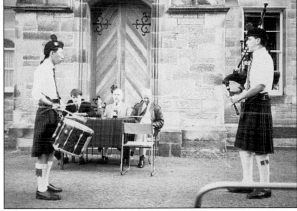

5.6 The value of large vital capacity.

The changing shape and size of children at puberty, resulting in alterations to the limb segments and the centre of mass of the body, may lead to technique breakdown in some early-age high skill sports such as gymnastics, trampolining, springboard and platform diving and ice-skating.

Lack of exercise may be more important than over-eating in many fat children, who have been shown to have lower calorie intakes than normal-weight controls.[16] Sixty percent of girls classed as overweight had daily intakes of less than 475kJ (2000kcal), while a similar percentage of normal-weight controls ingested 600kJ (2500kcal) daily.

Aerobic (cardiorespiratory) aspects

Respiratory parameters (**5.5**), such as vital capacity and FEV_1, are much the same in both sexes before puberty; vital capacity is significantly correlated with body height in children and adolescents.

Large vital capacity (**5.6**) may facilitate the playing of certain musical instruments, but it does not correlate highly with maximal oxygen uptake when correct scaling procedures are used to normalise the data. The peripheral aspects of aerobic fitness in children (muscle capillaries, myoglobin and mitochondria) may be increased by training. Centrally, however, lung volume increments are part of the growth in body dimensions, and are not dependent on training.[1]

In absolute terms, maximal oxygen uptake $\dot{V}O_2$(max) (**5.7**), is much the same in both sexes between the ages of five and 10, then girls gain a temporary advantage due to their earlier growth spurt. Typical values would be 47.8ml O_2.kg^{-1}.min^{-1} and 39.5ml O_2.kg^{-1}.min^{-1} for 12.8-year-old boys and girls respectively[3]. Between 16 and 19 years, typical values are 51.7 and 40.0ml O_2.kg^{-1}.min^{-1} respectively.[2] A study on runners at 800m to 3000m in this age-group[7] recorded mean $\dot{V}O_2$(max) values of 70.0ml O_2.kg^{-1}.min^{-1} in the boys, and 64.0ml in the girls.

Aerobic endurance training has the potential to control cardiac risk factors in schoolchildren[35] and may have therapeutic value in common diseases of childhood, such as asthma, cerebral palsy, cystic fibrosis, diabetes mellitus, myopathies and obesity.[31] The development of aerobic sports performance and the attack on cardiac risk factors may begin before puberty. If the type of programme recommended for the development of endurance fitness in adults is continued for 12 weeks or more, the $\dot{V}O_2$(max) of the prepubescent child is increased by about 15%, much as would be anticipated in an older person. The main mechanism for this gain appears to be an increase in stroke volume.

Systolic blood pressure during dynamic (as opposed to isometric) exercise in 500 healthy 9- to 18-year-olds showed higher elevations of pressure after puberty than before.[36] At heart rates of 170 beats per minute, 22 of the post-pubertal children reached systolic pressures of 200mmHg, with three at 240mm. Ice-skaters between 9 and 14 showed a

5.7

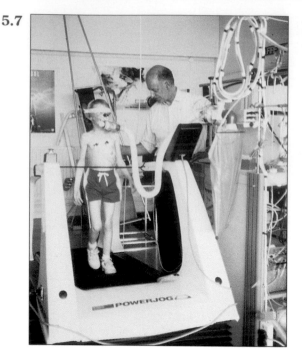

5.7 $\dot{V}O_2$(max) assessment

5.8

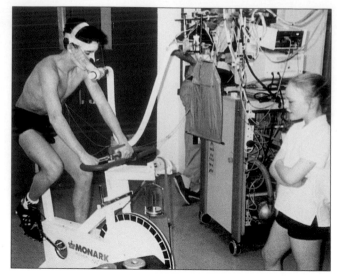

5.8 Cycle ergometry.

5.9

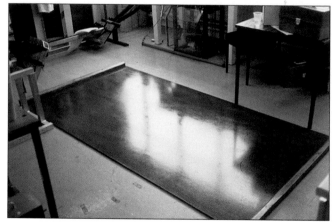

5.9 An ice-rink in the lab.

significant decrease in diastolic pressure, compared to controls.[20] These skaters trained more than 15 hours per week, with consequent improved vaso-pressor responses to exercise.

In general, at equivalent proportions of $\dot{V}O_2$(max), children's heart rates are approximately 20 beats.min^{-1} higher than adults. Significant cardiac dilatation and hypertrophy may occur in children before puberty after months of intense dynamic training, with corresponding regression on stopping training[14].

Cycle ergometry (**5.8**) is often considered to be the most accurate method of assessing $\dot{V}O_2$(max) in children, although it gives values approximately 5% less than the treadmill, due to utilisation of a lower percentage of muscle mass. Also, the cycle is more appropriate for some activities (judo, cycling, dance).

For endurance testing of young speed skaters, one can use a highly polished surface (**5.9**), such as the skaters may use in training. The subject performs the skating action in socks, at progressively increasing stride rates.

For young rowers, it is necessary to measure oxygen uptake during an exercise regime, such as rowing ergometry (**5.10**), which simulates the rowing action by using all four limbs.

For young canoeists, treadmill or cycle ergo-metery would test the wrong half of the body, so various forms of kayak or canoe ergometer are used (**5.11**).

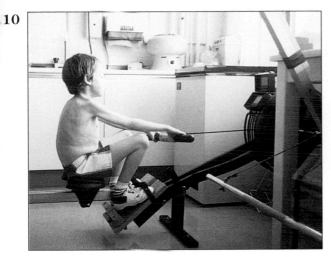

5.10

5.10 Rowing ergometry.

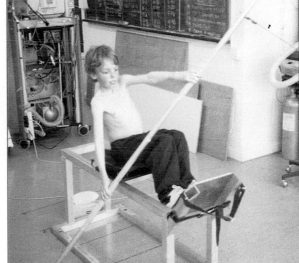

5.11

5.11 Kayak ergometry.

During exercise, children exhibit higher respiratory rates than adults, e.g. 60.min⁻¹ compared with 40.min⁻¹, at equivalent exercise levels. Also, the ventilatory equivalent for oxygen is greater, the younger the child[41] (**5.12**). Thus, per litre of oxygen, a six-year-old may need to ventilate 38 litres of air, compared to 28 litres at the age of 16. Apart from being modestly wasteful of energy, this may, especially in the younger child in a hot environment, induce hyperventilation hypocapnia, which is associated with dizziness and lightheadedness, together with paraesthesia of the lips and extremities, and even tetany, with lip stiffness and carpo-pedal spasm.

Tetany is usually ascribed to a low calcium ion concentration in blood and tissue fluids. In hyperventilation tetany, the total blood calcium is normal, but the calcium ionic fraction is increased due to the increase in calcium proteinate formation induced by the respiratory alkalosis. Treatment consists of short periods of re-breathing, using a medium-sized paper bag, for a few minutes. A recent report[10] recorded three cases in 13-year-old rugby players, in the same area, over a period of a few months.

Regarding the effectiveness of endurance training on prepubescent children (**5.13**), a recent review[31] lists a number of well-designed studies which show a positive response in such children, but to a lesser degree than in older subjects. Nevertheless, a seven-year-old is reported[25] to have covered the full marathon distance in under three and a half hours (which the author would certainly not advocate).

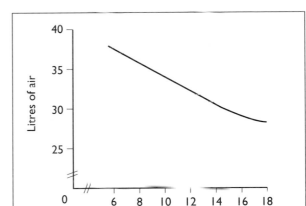

5.12

5.12 Maximum ventilatory equivalent (litres of air ventilated per litre of oxygen utilised) and age.

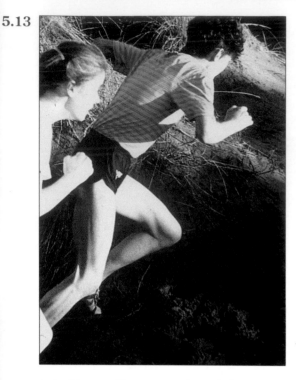

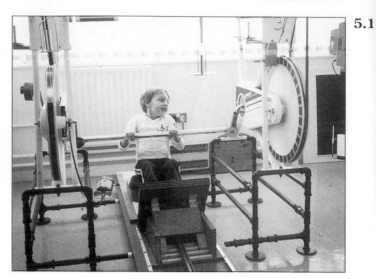

5.14 Supra-maximal anaerobic testing – upper body.

5.13 Young elite runners in training.

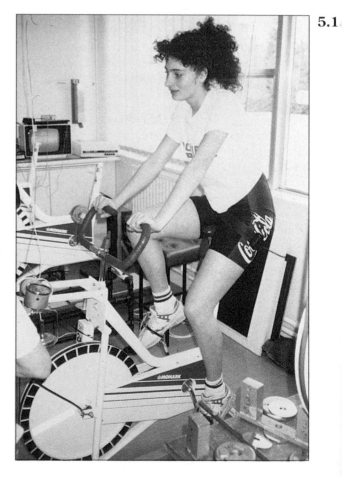

Elite competitors between the ages of 15 and 17 tend to show functional cardiac adaptations, with an accelerated myocardial hypertrophy occurring in their next three years.[27] Physical activity intense enough to increase aerobic fitness in prepubescent children appears to increase $\dot{V}O_2$(max) rather than the lactate threshold[4]. This is to be expected, as such children rely less on anaerobic glycolysis for energy production.

Anaerobic aspects – local muscle endurance

Some anaerobic parameters (power, endurance) of the upper and lower body (**5.14, 5.15**) may be measured by computing the velocity of an ergo-meter flywheel at frictional resistances appropriate to age, sex and sport, with peak and mean power, and rate of fatigue, results displayed in watts, and total work done in kJ. Most variants of this test last thirty seconds.

5.15 Top class young squash player performing anaerobic lower body test.

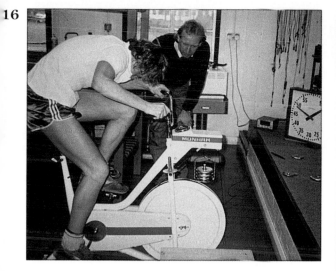

5.16 Anaerobic recovery testing.

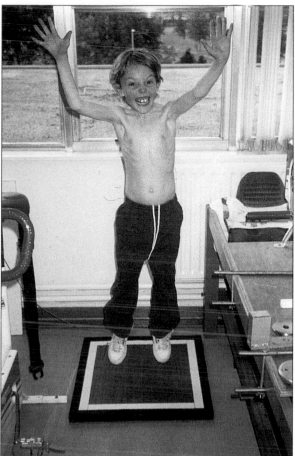

5.17 Another anaerobic power and endurance test.

Squash and other 'multiple sprint sport' players (badminton, hockey, lacrosse, shinty, hurling, camogie, gaelic football, soccer and rugby) repeat the anaerobic test four minutes later to assess the vital attribute of short term recovery (**5.16**).

In another anaerobic power and endurance test (**5.17**), the subject jumps continuously off a pressure mat for 30 or 60 seconds. The longer the off-the-mat time, as a proportion of the total, the greater the anaerobic endurance.

The ability of prepubescent children to perform anaerobic work is distinctly lower than that of adolescents, whose ability, in turn, is lower than adults.[17,30,40] Children have a much lower oxygen deficit, in proportion, than adults in the first few minutes of exercise, and gain their 'second wind' more quickly.[18] Their post-exercise oxygen consumption ('oxygen debt') is also less. Children seem to have lower levels of muscle glycogen, and appear to use lower proportions of it. Also, their rate of anaerobic glycolysis is lower, probably due to

lower levels of the rate-limiting glycolytic enzyme, phosphofructokinase.[9,12]

At equivalent percentages of their $\dot{V}O_2(max)$, children have lower levels of lactate the younger they are, e.g. approximately 50–60% of the adult level in 14-year-old boys.[8,12] Thus, children do not attain levels of acidosis as high as adolescents or adults. Irrespective of absolute values, there is an age-related change in maximal acidosis[19] at the decreasing rate of 0.01–0.02 pH units.year^{-1}.

The net result of all this is that children do not have the same fatigue barrier to vigorous exercise as adolescents or adults, which makes it easier for coaches or parents, unwittingly, to push them too hard in training sessions.

Nevertheless, boys between 11 and 15 years (and presumably girls) have been shown able to increase all their anaerobic parameters - including muscle glycogen concentration and utilisation rate, PFK activity, and anaerobic power – by appropriate interval training.[6,9,26]

5.18

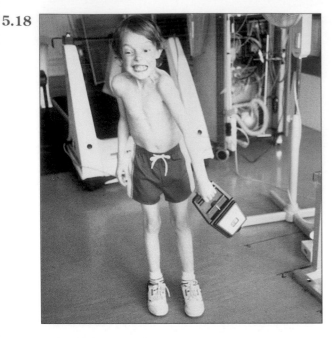

5.18 Grip strength assessed by a hand dynamo-meter.

5.1

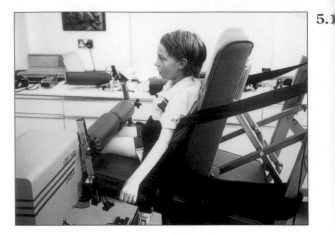

5.19 Isokinetic dynamometry for assessing force at given velocities of contraction.

5.2

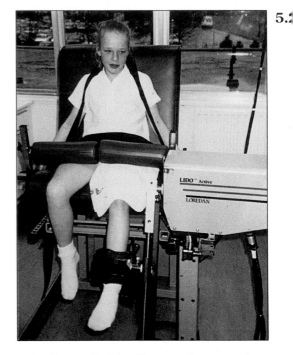

5.20 Emma Reid, elite ice skater under-going quadriceps and hamstring strength testing.

Strength

Strength can be measured in several different ways. Grip strength is assessed using a hand dynamo-meter (**5.18**). Quadriceps and hamstring force production is estimated at different contraction velocities on an isokinetic dynamometer (**5.19, 5.20**). Strength of the back and abdomen is important in many sports, especially rowing and gymnastics (**5.21**). Strain gauge dynamometry is simpler (and many times cheaper) than isokinetic devices and can be useful. In **5.22**, isometric assessment of back strength is being made on young elite rowers.

For young children, strength training is most safely done utilising the child's own body weight as the resistance (**5.23**).

In prepubescents, 25–35% of their body mass is muscle, which increases after puberty to 40-45% in boys, and 35–38% in girls. The sex difference is due partly to increased female body-fat, and partly to androgen stimulation being greater in males.[37] Strength increases naturally with growth, probably reaching a peak during the adolescent growth spurt in girls, and a year after in boys.[24]

Suitable progressive resistance training will increase strength in girls[22] and boys.[23,38] Until full

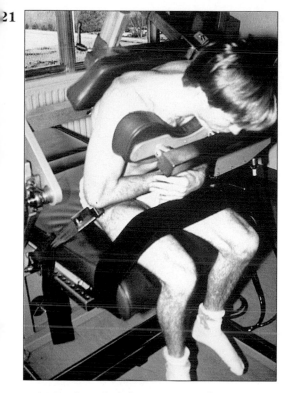

5.21 Back and abdomen strength testing.

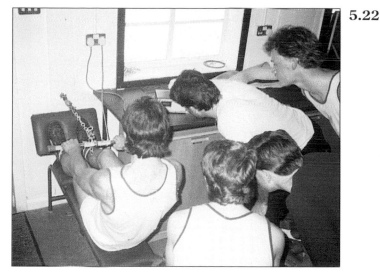

5.22 Strain gauge dynamometry.

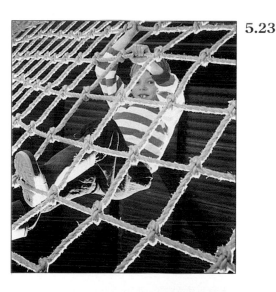

5.23 Body-weight strength training.

bone growth has been reached, it is advisable to limit heavy resistance training. Certainly, pre-pubescents should be restricted to utilising their body weight for strength training. Even then, deep squats, extensor thrusts against resistance and injudicious plyometric work may induce muscle injury and bone damage.[13]

Force production, per given area, of children's muscle is similar to adults.[8] However, the relative *power* of children's muscle increases with age (**5.24**), through greater myofibrillar density, increases in contraction velocity and development of neuromuscular transmission.[28] When longitudinal growth stops, adults continue to increase the cross-sectional area of muscle, possibly changing the angle of pennation and giving better mechanical advantage.[29]

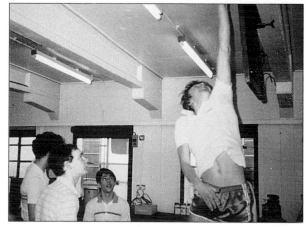

5.24. The vertical jump test. The use of body weight and the Lewis nomogram renders it a useful test of leg power.

5.25

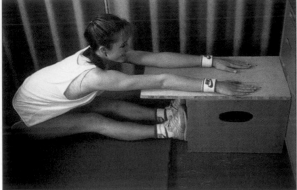

5.

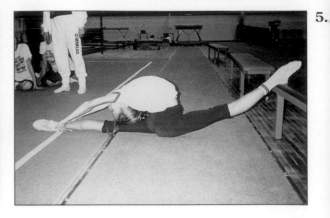

5.25 Hamstring and lower lumbar flexibility measurement.

5.26 Sports-specific flexibility testing (gymnastics).

5.

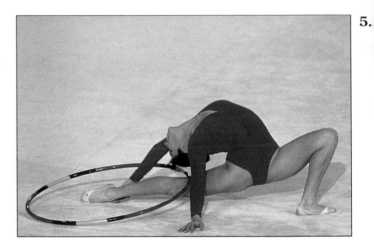

5.27 Flexibility in action, in rhythmic gymnastics.

Flexibility

There are simple tests for measuring hamstring and lower lumbar flexibility (**5.25**), and others for specifically measuring gymnastic flexibility (**5.26**).

Much of the flexibility in gymnastics, trampolining, diving and dance involves the active range of movement (**5.27**). This often requires considerable strength to attain and hold the position and such muscular strength also serves to stabilise the joint. Flexibility usually decreases with growth, especially during the growth spurt, when the increased length of bone stretches the attached muscles. Poor flexibility may be an important cause of over-use injuries.[5,13,15] Slow, static (non-ballistic) stretching, preceded by a warm-up, is most suitable for children. The muscle should be slowly stretched, and held for about 10 seconds, about five times alternately on each side.

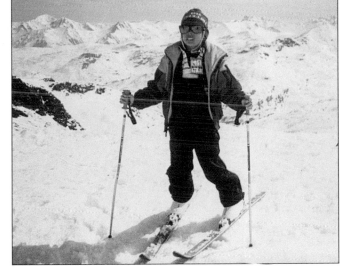

5.29, 5.30 Laboratory balance tests are useful in appropriate sports.

5.28 The stabilometer.

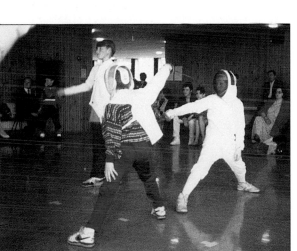

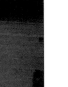

Balance and coordination

The stabilometer is an electronic see-saw which provides data on balance and coordination (**5.28**). Children generally have a better sense of balance than adults, partly due to their smaller body size and lower centre of mass.

Laboratory balance tests are useful in sports such as skiing (**5.29**), and also in fencing (**5.30**), canoeing, rowing, shooting, archery, board-sailing, squash and badminton.

The 'extreme balance' activities such as gymnastics, dance and platform diving tend to have their own sports-specific balance tests (**5.31**).

5.31 Sports-specific balance testing (gymnastics).

5.32

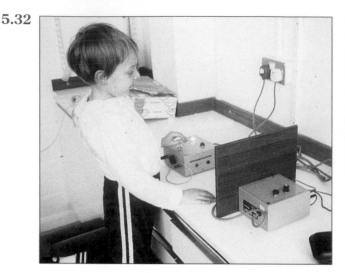

5.32 Response testing.

5.

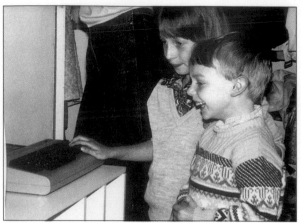

5.33 Enjoying the test.

Reactions

Fast responses and quick movements are essential components of most sporting activities. Their evaluation (**5.32**) is important in possible talent identification and in monitoring training . Auditory and visual response times both tend to decrease reasonably linearly from around 400msec at the age of five, to about 200msec at 15, with the auditory response consistently being the faster by some 40-50msec.[33] Generally, children particularly enjoy auditory or visual response tests (**5.33**).

Nature versus nurture?

The child featured in **5.34** is the son of two international competitors; the father a distance runner and the mother a squash player who represented her country over 70 times. Bearing in mind that all mitochondria are maternally derived, that genetic coding of neural organisation for visual tasks dependent on the manipulation of spatial relationships (e.g. as in racket and ball skills) may be located on the X-chromosome as recessive factors; and that scientific papers are beginning to be published with titles stressing the inheritance of the ability to respond to training[32], it could become increasingly important for coaches to assess parents (especially mothers) in selecting youngsters for advanced training. This indeed has been the practice in some sports in Eastern Europe for many years.

5.

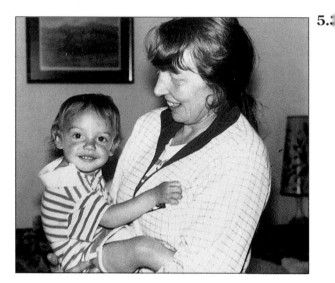

5.34 Winning genes?

If children play a sport themselves, then they appreciate watching it all the more (**5.35**), and in this manner, learn to play it better. It is to be hoped that they increase their enjoyment in both spectating and participating. Sport, and especially children's sport, should be fun.

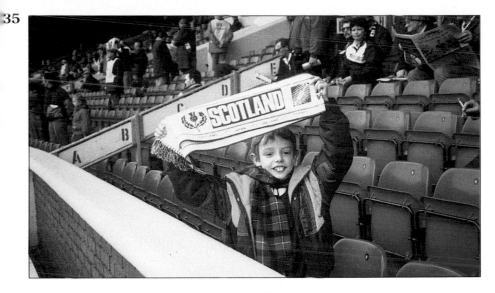

5.35 A keen young spectator (at Murrayfield).

Acknowledgements

Illustrations **5.3**, **5.4**, **5.7** and **5.18** are courtesy of Vivian Grisogono; **5.13** is courtesy of Leo Faulmann; **5.26** and **5.31** are courtesy of Sarah Wykeham; and **5.27** is courtesy of Bob Martin, Allsport, to all of whom I tender my most grateful thanks. I am also very grateful to Duncan McNeill Sharp for his patience and enthusiasm in the laboratory in allowing us to photograph him under test. Many thanks should be accorded to the other recorded subjects including the Pipes and Drums of Morrison's Academy, Crieff. Special thanks are due to Vivian Grisogono for her general expert and generous help, and to Dr Nicola Maffulli for his generosity of mind.

References

1. Andersen, K.L., Rutenfranz, J., Ilmarinen, J. *et al.* (1983) The growth of lung volumes affected by physical performance capacity in boys and girls during adolescence and childhood. *Eur. J. App. Physiol. and Occup. Physiol.* **52(4)**: 380–384.
2. Anderson, L.B., Henckel, P. and Saltin, B. (1987) Maximal oxygen uptake in Danish adolescents 16–19 years of age. *Eur. J. App. Physiol. and Occup. Physiol.* **56(1)**: 74-82.
3. Armstrong, N., Balding, J., Gentle, P. and Kirby, B. (1990) Estimation of risk factors for chronic disease in children from 15 countries. *Prev. Med.* **10**:121–132.
4. Atomi, Y., Iwaoka, K., Hatta, H., Myashita, M. and Yamamoto, Y. (1986) Daily physical activity levels in pre-adolescent boys related to VO_2(max) and lactate thresholds. *Eur. J. App. Physiol. and Occup. Physiol.* **55(2)**: 151–161.
5. Beck, J.L. and Day, R.W. (1985) Overuse injuries. *Clin. Sports Med.* **4(3)**: 553–573.
6. Cunningham, D.A. and Patterson, D.H. (1988) Physiological characteristics of young active boys. In: Brown, E.W. and Branta, C.F. (Eds) *Competitive Sports for Children and Youth*, pp. 159–169. Human Kinetics Publishers, Champaign, Ill.
7. Davies, C.T.M. (1982) Aerobic performance in young children. In: Russo, P.S. and Gass, G. (Eds) *Children and Exercise: a Conference*, pp. 42–45. Cumberland College of Health Sciences, Sydney, NSW.
8. Davies, C.T.M. (1985) Strength and mechanical properties of muscle in children and young adults. *Scand. J. Sports Sci.* **7(1)**: 11–15.
9. Eriksson, B.O., Karlsson, J. and Saltin, B. (1971) Muscle metabolites during exercise in pubertal boys. *Acta Paediatr. Scand. Suppl.* **217**: 154–157.
10. Flanagan, M. (1992) Hyperventilation. *Sports Med. and Soft Tissue Trauma (Lederle)*, **4(2)**: 16.
11. Frisch, R.E. (1984) Body fat, puberty and fertility. *Biol. Rev. (London)*, **59(2)**, 161–188.
12. Fournier, M., Ricci, J., Taylor, A.W. *et al.* (1982) Skeletal muscle adaptation in adolescent boys: sprint and endurance training and detraining. *Med. Sci. Sports and Exerc.* **14**: 453–456.
13. Grisogono, V. (1991) In: *Children and Sport: Fitness, Injuries and Diet*, Ch. 7,8 and 9. John Murray, London.
14. Hanne-Paparo, N. (1987) The athlete's heart: a review. *Int. J. Sports Cardiol. (Turin)* **4(1)**: 47–57.
15. Highgenbotom, C.L. (1981) Children's knee problems. *Orthop. Rev.* **10**: 37–48.
16. Johnson, M.L., Burke, B.S. and Mayer, J. Relative importance of inactivity and overeating in the energy balance of obese high school girls. *Am. J. Clin. Nutr.* **4**: 37–44.

17. Kurowski, T.T. (1983) Anaerobic power of children from ages 9 through 15 years. MSc Thesis, Florida State University. Quoted in Bar-Or *Pediatric Sports Medicine for the Practitioner*, pp. 11–12. Springer-Verlag, NY.

18. Macek, M. and Vavra, J. (1980) The adjustments of oxygen uptake at the onset of exercise: a comparison between pre-pubertal boys and young adults. *Int. J. Sports Med.* **1**: 75–77.

19. Matějková", J., Kopřivová, Z. and Placheta, Z. (1980) Changes in acid-base balance after maximal exercise. In: Placheta, Z. (Ed.) *Youth and Physical Activity*, pp. 191–199. J.E.Purkyne University, Brno.

20. Michel-Panichi, C., Mandel, C., Auriacombe, L., Pedroni, E., Kachaner, J. and Hennequet, A. (1987) Echocardiography in children practising ice-skating. *Med. du Sport (Paris)* **61(3)**: 159–163.

21. Nevill, A., Ramsbottom, R. and Williams, C. (1992) Scaling physiological measurements for individuals of different body size. *Eur.J. Appl. Physiol.* In Press.

22. Nielsen, B., Nielsen, K., Behrendt-Hansen, M. and Asmussen, E. (1980) Training of functional strength in girls 7-19 years old. In: Berg, K. and Erikson, B. (Eds) *Children and Exercise IX*, pp. 68–69. University Park Press, Baltimore.

23. Pfeiffer, R. and Francis, R.S. (1986) Effects of strength training on muscle development in pre-pubescent, pubescent and post-pubescent males. *Phys. Sportsmed.* **14**: 134–136.

24. Potthast, J. and Klimt, F. (1988) Vertical power measurements of selected leg power exercises using capacitative measuring platforms. *Deut. Zeit. Sportmed. (Cologne)* **39(8)**: 300–306.

25. Roberts, R. (1982) Marathon running and children. In: Russo, P.S. and Gass, G. (Eds) *Children and Exercise: a Conference*, pp. 51–55. Cumberland College of Health Sciences, Sydney, NSW.

26. Rotstein, A., Dotan, R., Bar-Or, O. and Tenenbaum, G. (1986) Effect of training on anaerobic threshold, maximal aerobic power and anaerobic performance of pre-adolescent boys. *Int. J. Sports Med.* **7**: 281–286.

27. Rusko, H. (1985) Youth and top-class sport: endurance training effects on young athletes. *Int. Council of Sports Sci. and Phys. Ed. Rev. (Berlin)* **8**: 54–64.

28. Sargeant, A.J. (1989) Short-term muscle power in children and adolescents. In: Bar-Or, O. (Ed.) *Advances in Pediatric Sports Sciences*, Vol. 3, pp. 41–66. Human Kinetics Publishers, Champaign, Ill.

29. Sargeant, A.J. and Dolan, P. (1986) Optimal velocity of muscle contraction for short-term power output (anaerobic) in children and adults. In: Rutenfranz, J., Mocellin, R. and Klimt, F. (Eds) *Children and Exercise XII*, pp. 39–42. Human Kinetics Publishers, Champaign, Ill.

30. Sargeant, A.J., Dolan, P. and Thorne, A. (1984) Isokinetic measurement of maximal force and anaerobic power in children. In: Ilimarinen, J. and Valimaki, I. (Eds) *Children and Sport*, pp. 93–98. Springer-Verlag, Berlin.

31. Shephard, R.J. (1992) Effectiveness of training programmes for pubescent children. *Sports Med.* **13(3)**: 194–231.

32. Simoneau, J.A., Lortie, G., Boulay, M.R., Marcotte, M., Thibault, M.C. and Bouchard, C. (1986) Inheritance of human skeletal muscle and anaerobic capacity adaptation to high intensity intermittent training. *Int. J. Sports Med.* **7(3)**: 167–171.

33. Szmodis, I., Szabo, T., Rendi, M., Temesi, Z. and Meszaros, Z. (1984) Performance in plate-tapping and simple reaction time of children aged 5–15 years. In: Ilimarinen, J. and Valimaki, I. (Eds) *Children and Sport*, pp. 42–45. Springer-Verlag, Berlin.

34. Tanner, J.M. (1949) Fallacy of per-weight and per-surface area standards and their relation to spurious correlation. *J. Appl. Physiol.* **2(1)**: 1–15.

35. Vaccaro, P. and Mahon, A.D. (1989) The effect of exercise on coronary heart disease risk factors in children. *Sports Med.* **8**: 139–153.

36. Wanne, O.P.S. and Haapoja, E. (1988) Blood pressure during exercise in healthy children. *Eur. J. Appl. Physiol. and Occup. Physiol.* **1/2**: 62–67.

37. Wells, C.L. (1985) The limits of female performance. In: Clarke, D.H. and Eckert, H.M. (Eds) *American Academy of Physical Education Papers* 18, pp. 81–92. Human Kinetics Publishers, Champaign, Ill.

38. Weltman. A., Janney, C., Rians, C.B. *et al.* (1986) The effects of hydraulic resistance strength training in pre-pubertal males. *Med. Sci. Sports Exerc.* **18(6)**: 629–638.

39. Williams, J.R., Armstrong, N., Winter, E.M. and Crichton, N. (1992) Changes in peak oxygen uptake with age and sexual maturation in boys: physiological fact or statistical anomaly. *Procs. 16th Pediatric Work Physiology Conference*, In Press. Clemont Ferrand.

40. Zwiren, L.D. (1989) Anaerobic and aerobic capacities of children. *Ped. Exerc. Sci.* **1(1)**: 31–44.

41. Bar-Or, O. (1983) *Pediatric Sports Medicine for the Practitioner*. Springer-Verlag Inc, New York.

Suggested reading

Armstrong, N., Balding, J. Gentle, P. and Kirby, B. (1990) Patterns of physical activity among 11–16 year old British children. *Br. Med. J.* **301**: 203–205.

Armstrong, N., Balding, J. Gentle, P. and Kirby, B. (1990) The estimation of coronary risk factors in British schoolchildren - a preliminary report. *Br. J. Sports Med.* **24**: 61–66.

Bale, P. (1992) The functional performance of children in relation to growth, maturation and exercise. *Sports Med.* **13(3)**: 151–159.

Falkner, F. and Tanner, J.M. (Eds) (1986) *Human Growth 2 - Postnatal Growth*. Plenum Press, NY.

Grisogono, V. (1991) *Children and Sport: Fitness, Injuries and Diet*. John Murray (Publishers) Ltd, London.

Maffulli,N. and Helms, P. (1988) Controversies about intensive training in young athletes. *Arch. Dis. Child.* **63**:1045–1047.

Maffulli, N.and Pintore E. (1990) Intensive training in young athletes. *Br. J. Sports Med.* **24**:237–239.

Maffulli, N. (1992) The growing child in sport. *Br Med Bull.* **48**:561–568.

6. Nutrition

Gabe Mirkin

The nutritional needs of children and adolescent athletes are the same as those for their adult counterparts. This chapter will review the physiological principles that can be used as a foundation for advising young athletes on how to use sound nutritional principles to maintain their health and maximise their performance in sports.

Nutrients

Humans require approximately 46 nutrients to be healthy (**Table 6.1**). Lack of even one nutrient can impair performance, but taking massive doses of any single nutrient will not improve performance.

How food is utilised by the body

Carbohydrates, proteins and fats are the only nutritional sources of energy. Before they can pass into the bloodstream, they must first be separated from other components of food and be catabolised into their basic building blocks: carbohydrates into single sugars, proteins into single and small chains of amino acids, and fats into monoglycerides, glycerol and fatty acids.

Only four sugars can pass into the bloodstream: glucose, fructose, galactose and mannose. The last three are immediately taken up by the liver and converted to the fourth, glucose. All cells can use glucose for energy. Glucose that is not used immediately can be stored only as glycogen – in muscle and liver cells. When these tissues are saturated with glycogen, all excess glucose is converted to triglycerides. Liver glycogen can be released into the bloodstream, while muscle glycogen can be utilised only by that specific muscle.

Most of the ingested protein is used to form structural components. It can also be used to supply as much as 15% of energy during exercise, with more than half coming from one amino acid, leucine. Most leucine does not come from ingested protein. The nitrogen comes from other branched-chain amino acids (isoleucine and valine) and most of the carbon comes from glucose and other amino acids. Before

Table 6.1. Table of nutrients.

Water

Linoleic acid

9 amino acids

13 vitamins

Approximately 21 minerals

Glucose (for energy)

amino acids can be used for energy, deamination and transamination must occur to remove the nitrogen.

Epithelial cells lining the intestines combine glycerol and fatty acids to form triglycerides which can be used immediately for energy or be stored for future use in fat, muscle and other cells.

Maximising endurance

Endurance is the ability to continue exercising muscles for an extended period of time. The major sources of energy are triglycerides and glycogen in muscles and triglycerides and glucose in blood. Most blood triglyceride comes from fat stores, whereas most blood glucose is synthesised by the liver.

There is a virtually unlimited amount of fat stored in the body. The fat cells of athletes contain enough fat to support exercise for 119 hours. However, muscles contain only enough glycogen to last one and a half hours, and the liver contains only enough glycogen to last six minutes. As exercise intensity increases, the percentage of energy from muscle glycogen also increases. When muscles become depleted of their glycogen, they hurt and become more difficult to coordinate. This is called 'hitting the wall'. No chemical explanation for this effect is evident.[1] The explanation that lack of glycogen causes fatigue by blocking the regeneration of ATP is not supported by experimental studies.

Low muscle glycogen levels cause only a minimal decrease in ATP levels. T.D. Noakes has shown that muscle fatigue during endurance events is caused more by damage to the muscle fibres themselves than by lack of available glycogen. Recent research shows that muscle endurance can be enhanced by strengthening muscle fibres by exercising them against increasing resistance. For a runner, skier, cycler, skater or swimmer, that means to exercise at a faster pace one to three times a week.

An athlete can increase endurance by:

- Maximising muscle glycogen prior to competition.
- Conserving glycogen by burning more fat (and less glycogen), eating food and drinking energy-rich fluids during competition.

Ninety-eight per cent of the energy for the brain comes from circulating blood glucose. However, there is only enough glucose in the blood to last three minutes at rest, so the liver must provide constant replacement. The liver contains enough glycogen to supply glucose for only six minutes, so it must constantly synthesise glucose from protein.

Most conditioned athletes can tolerate low blood sugar levels during exercise without experiencing untoward effects.[2] However, when blood levels of glucose fall below 30mg/dl, some can feel tired or dizzy and even suffer a syncopal episode. This is called 'bonking'. Bicyclists who do not eat during endurance races may experience this after four or more hours of racing.

Athletes can increase endurance prior to competition by:

- Using special training methods.
- Manipulating their diet.

During competition, endurance can be increased by:

- Taking in additional foods and supplements.
- Using certain techniques such as starting out slowly.
- Maintaining a relatively constant intensity.
- Choosing mid-temperature and low-humidity weather.

Training to increase endurance

To increase glycogen stores in muscle and conserve available glycogen, athletes preparing for endurance events utilise a training technique called depletion.[3] Once a week, to deplete muscle glycogen stores, they exercise for an extended period after their muscles ache and feel heavy. This increases production of muscle glycogen synthetase.[4] When depletion training is done more often, recovery is delayed, restricting the amount of intense training that can be done during the rest of the week.

As described in the previous section, intense training also helps to increase endurance. Most athletes in endurance sports set up their weekly training programmes to include two very intense workouts to strengthen muscle fibres and one extended workout to deplete muscle glycogen **(Table 6.2)**.

Table 6.2 World-class marathon runners' endurance programme.

	Type of workout	Example
Monday	easy	jog 6–10 miles
Tuesday	intense	short intervals: run 100 very fast 15–30 sec runs, each followed by slow jogging until recovery occurs
Wednesday	easy	jog 6–10 miles
Thursday	intense	long intervals: run six 800m repeats at 95% effort with a 400m jog between each
Friday	day off	rest
Saturday	easy	jog 10 miles
Sunday	long	90–120 mins running at a steady pace

Eating to increase endurance

When athletes ingest more food than their body can utilise at that time, the extra nutrients are stored as glycogen in the liver and muscle. When these stores are filled, the liver converts all extra calories to fat which is then stored in the body. Extra fat creates extra weight which can slow the athlete during competition. Any dietary manipulation that advocates increased energy intake or decreased energy expenditure for more than three days will usually increase fat stores.

Eating during the week before competition

In 1939, Swedish researchers showed that a high carbohydrate diet will increase muscle glycogen stores.[5] In the mid 1960s, Per Olof Astrand recommended the following dietary manoeuvre.[6] Seven days prior to competition, an athlete should perform a long depletion workout. For the next three days, he keeps the glycogen content of his muscles low by eating a very low carbohydrate diet. For the next three days, he eats his regular diet plus extra carbohydrate-rich foods (**Table 6.3**).

Most top athletes have abandoned this regimen because more recent research shows that athletes can load their muscles maximally with glycogen just by markedly reducing their workouts for the three days prior to competition. A further limitation of the regimen is that athletes cannot train effectively during the depletion phase. Furthermore, the ingestion of very large amounts of carbohydrates has been reported to cause chest pain,[7] myoglobinuria and nephritis.[8] For six days prior to major competitions, most athletes restrict intense workouts and for three days prior to competition, they eat their regular meals plus a little extra carbohydrate.[9]

Table 6.4 High-carbohydrate foods for the 'last supper.'

High-Fat Meal

Pasta with Tomato Sauce and Meatballs
  or Pizza
Milk
Juice
Garlic Bread
Apple Pie

or

Low-Fat Meal

Large Vegetable Salad
Bean and Eggplant (aubergene) Casserole
Bread
Rolls
Juice
Fruit

Table 6.3 High-carbohydrate foods.

Pasta
Fruits
Vegetables
Beans
Grains and Cereals
Most Bakery Goods
Confectionery
Desserts

Eating the night before competition

For his 'last supper', the athlete usually eats a high-carbohydrate meal (**Table 6.4**). This helps to maximise muscle glycogen stores. The pre-game meal cannot serve this function since it takes at least 10 hours to replenish muscle glycogen.[10] The meal can contain either simple sugars or complex carbohydrates or any combination of each. It can be either high or low in fat, and it should contain fibre to facilitate evacuation.

Eating the pre-competition meal

The athlete can eat anything that he wants before a competition, provided that it will pass through the stomach by the time the competition starts. A high-fat meal has not been shown to increase endurance by causing muscles to utilise increased amounts of fat with resultant sparing of muscle glycogen. A high-sugar meal has not been shown to decrease endurance by increasing muscle utilisation of glycogen. Fructose offers no advantage over glucose. Glycerol solutions, ingested either before or during exercise, have not been shown to increase endurance or hydration or to improve tolerance to exercise in the heat.[11]

The pre-competition meal should be eaten not more than five hours prior to competition. Liver glycogen is necessary to maintain blood glucose levels. There is only enough glycogen in hepatocytes to last twelve hours when the athlete is at rest.[12] If more than a few hours elapse between the pre-competition meal and the time of competition, considerable amounts of liver glycogen will be catabolised. Eating replenishes liver glycogen stores. The athlete can eat right up to the time of competition if that meal can pass from his stomach by the time he starts to compete.

Eating during competition

Most athletes do not need to eat during events lasting fewer than two hours. However, in events lasting longer than that, athletes can benefit from ingesting additional food or drinking fluids that contain carbohydrates. The fitter an athlete, the better he is able to utilise ingested carbohydrates during exercise.[13]

One of the leading researchers on energy requirements during exercise is Dr. David Costill of Ball State University in Muncie, Indiana. He feels that to enhance endurance, the very least amount of carbohydrate that increases endurance is $40g.hour^{-1}$. Optimum is closer to twice that level. That would explain why bicycle racers eat solid foods during competition. Otherwise, they would have to drink at least 800ml of a 10% carbohydrate drink per hour. This would pose a problem because only 600ml can pass through the stomach in one hour.

Athletes should eat small amounts of carbohydrate-rich foods frequently, rather than large amounts occasionally. There is less variation in blood sugar levels and enhanced sprint performance at the end of competition.[14] While optimum frequency has not been determined, it may be prudent to eat 10g of carbohydrate every 15 minutes or 20g every 30 minutes (**Table 6.5**).

Drinking during training

During training, particularly in hot weather, some athletes become increasingly dehydrated and suffer progressive weakness and deterioration in performance. Thirst is not a dependable signal of dehydration. To prevent dehydration during early season workouts in hot weather, the athlete should be weighed before and after practice. For every 1/2 kilogram that he loses, he needs to ingest 500ml of fluids immediately after practice.

Table 6.5 Examples of easily digested foods to be eaten during competition.

	grams of carbohydrate
1 slice bread	13
1 water bagel	30
4 graham crackers	21
1 fig bar	11
1 orange	16
1 cup grapes	20
1 banana	26

Drinking before competition

Although most athletes do not benefit from eating in events that last fewer than two hours, virtually all benefit from maintaining hydration. Competitive athletes can lose up to two $litres.hour^{-1}$ of fluid during intense exercise in warm weather. The maximum rate of stomach emptying is $600ml.hour^{-1}$ ($10ml.minute^{-1}$). Therefore, no matter how much fluid athletes ingest during competition, they will not be able to replenish their fluid losses completely during intense exercise.

An athlete can increase hydration during the week prior to competition and immediately before competition. Doubling the athlete's daily intake of fluid for one week, from one litre to two, can increase blood volume by 10%. The extra fluid is not lost completely as urine.[15]

After fluid leaves the stomach, it is absorbed almost immediately. The only way to increase the rate that water is absorbed is to make it leave the stomach faster. Nancy Rehrer of the University of Limberg in the Netherlands has shown that filling the stomach with water markedly accelerates stomach emptying.[16]

If athletes drink a large amount of water a half hour before competition, they will start a race with full bladders. However, if they drink 600ml of water just before the race starts, their stomachs will be full and their bladders will be empty. Almost 400ml will pass into the intestines in 20 minutes.[17] Thereafter, they should try to ingest 142ml of water every 10 minutes.

Drinking during competition

Athletes should drink before they feel thirsty. They do not feel thirsty until they have lost one to two litres of fluid. By that time, performance is compromised and fluid cannot be completely replaced. The athlete loses water during exercise primarily through sweating. Sweat contains a far lower concentration of salt than blood. Therefore, athletes lose far more water than salt, causing the concentration of salt in the blood to rise. A person will not feel thirsty until the concentration of salt in the blood rises to the level at which the thirst osmoreceptors in the brain are activated.

What to drink

Many athletes prefer to drink water for exercise that lasts less than one hour.[18,19] However, athletes who exercise longer than that also need energy sources and minerals. The rules for energy-containing fluids have changed dramatically in the last few years. In 1968, studies showed that 2.5% was the highest concentration of sugar that could be contained in an exercise drink and still be absorbed.[20] This posed a problem because drinks taste best when they contain a 10% concentration of sugar. Soft drinks and fruit juices contain 10% sugar. Soon after these studies, many exercise drinks containing 2.5% appeared on the market. They did not taste good because the concentration of sugar was too low, so some of the manufacturers added saccharin to sweeten the taste.

Twenty years later, new studies refuted the 1968 report. The 1968 data were collected on resting subjects. Exercise increases gastric emptying for both solid meals and liquids.[21] When the same studies were repeated using people who were exercising at an intense level, 10% sugared drinks were absorbed rapidly. Based on the most recent evidence, special exercise drinks are not necessary, although many athletes may prefer them. All 10% drinks are equally effective in supplying energy (**Table 6.6**). This recent data seems to conflict with previous data showing the need for special drinks that contain polymers of five glucose molecules bound together. Polymers are supposed to provide a high percentage of sugar at a low osmotic pressure, thereby not delaying absorption. However, they are not superior to free glucose for maintaining hydration and blood glucose levels, and they have not been shown to increase endurance.[22]

Electrolytes

Additional minerals are not needed in exercise that takes less than two hours. Sweat is so dilute, when compared to blood, that blood levels of sodium and potassium rise during exercise, calcium stays the same, and only magnesium levels drop. However, this drop in the blood level of magnesium is caused by that ion leaving the bloodstream to enter red blood cells.[23]

Dilute mineral drinks may be necessary to improve performance in events lasting longer than three hours (**Table 6.7**). As long as they are hypotonic in comparison to blood, they are absorbed almost as rapidly as pure water.[24] Recent research shows that the sucrose concentration of a drink affects absorption far more than its sodium concentration. Sodium also increases sugar absorption. Hypertonic drinks markedly delay stomach emptying.[25] However, athletes need extra calories during events lasting longer than three hours and, in these events, most athletes replace their minerals by eating solid food.

Cold or warm, with bubbles or without? (**Table 6.8**). In the 1960s, data showed that cold drinks (4°C) are absorbed faster than warm ones. The theory was that cold water causes the stomach to contract and push fluids rapidly into the intestines.

Table 6.6 To make a 10% sugared drink.

Dissolve 8 tablespoons of sugar in one litre of water

1 tablespoon contains 12 grams of sucrose

Table 6.7 Optimal mineral content of drinks for competition.

	(mg per litre)
Sodium	400–1,100
Chloride	500–1,500
Potassium	120–224
Calcium	45–225
Magnesium	10–100[26]

Table 6.8 Drinks for competition.

Most carbonated soft drinks
Most fruit juices
5–10% sugared water or tea

However, more recent studies show that temperature does not make much difference.[27,28] Furthermore, carbonated drinks are absorbed as rapidly as non-carbonated ones.[29]

Eating and drinking after competition

Much of post-competition tiredness is caused by depletion of body water and muscle glycogen. It makes no difference whether the carbohydrate replenishment is with simple sugars found in fruits or more complex sugars found in grains and beans. The average athlete takes in 250 grams of carbohydrate each day. He can maximise recovery by taking in three times that for one or two days.[30]

The timing and amount of carbohydrate intake also significantly affect glycogen replenishment. Two hours after competition, athletes who ate immediately had three times as much muscle glycogen as those who ate nothing.[31] Furthermore, the maximal amount of glycogen replenishment comes from eating 225 grams of carbohydrate (**Table 6.9**). Eating more carbohydrate than that does not increase further the rate of glycogen replenishment.[32]

Table 6.9 225-gram carbohydrate post-exercise meal.	
2 rolls, each with	
3 tablespoons of jam	120 grams
2 bananas	60
2 cups orange juice	52
Total	232

The athlete's diet

To meet energy needs, athletes should obtain 55 to 70% of their calories from carbohydrates, rather than the 45% of the average sedentary person. The average person ingests 38% of calories from fat. This high-fat intake is associated with an increased risk of developing coronary artery disease and cancers of the prostate, breast, uterus, colon and gall bladder. For health reasons only, it appears to be prudent to reduce fat intake to 10–20% of calories, leaving 10–15 for protein.

There is some evidence that an extremely low-fat diet (fewer than $20g.day^{-1}$) during growth can limit ultimate adult height. There is no evidence that a 10% fat diet will interfere with growth when caloric intake is high.

A simple way to obtain a 70/20/10 ratio is to eat two thirds carbohydrate-rich food and one third protein-rich food. To maintain muscle glycogen, athletes in endurance sports, such as long distance running, cycling and skiing, need to take in at least 600 grams of carbohydrate each day. Otherwise, they will suffer from fatigue and a drop in training performance. Athletes should eat a wide variety of high-carbohydrate foods, complemented with a lesser amount of high-protein foods.

Athletes need vitamins and minerals. With the exception of calcium and iron, mineral deficiencies rarely occur in athletes. Iron levels can be checked by measuring serum ferritin. Low iron reserves, even in the absence of anaemia, can interfere with lactic acid clearance during exercise.[33] If low, daily iron supplements or a high meat-fish-chicken diet may be prescribed. Iron tablets should not be prescribed to athletes who are not deficient in that mineral. Excesssive iron intake can cause zinc deficiency[34] and damage to internal organs.

Amaenorrhic female athletes may need to take in 1500mg of calcium each day, instead of the usual 1000mg. They can do this by taking in extra high-calcium foods (**Table 6.10**) or by taking calcium supplements.

Even though athletes have increased needs for thiamine, niacin, riboflavin and pantothenic acid they receive ample supplies from the vast amount of food that they eat and rarely suffer from vitamin deficiencies. Most vitamins are parts of enzymes which are continuously recycled and therefore are not used up in energy production. Even though a varied diet should supply all of the necessary vitamins, it is perfectly safe for an athlete to take a supplement containing the recommended dietary allowances for vitamins.

A simple guide for healthful eating is the four-food plan (**Table 6.11**). A well-balanced diet should contain at least eight servings of the first two groups and three servings of the last two. This should supply adequate amounts of vitamins.

Table 6.10 Foods that contain 250mg of calcium.
1 glass milk (240ml)
1 cup yogurt (120ml)
1 1/2 cups cottage cheese
1 1/2 cups ice cream
1 1/2 slices hard cheese
2 ounces sardines with bones
4 ounces canned salmon with bones
1 250 mg calcium carbonate pill

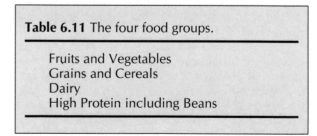

Table 6.11 The four food groups.
Fruits and Vegetables
Grains and Cereals
Dairy
High Protein including Beans

Losing weight

The most effective way for most athletes and regular exercisers to lose weight is to increase the intensity and duration of their workouts without altering their diets. However, some athletes cannot lose weight unless they also manipulate their diets.

Calorie restriction is rarely an effective means for athletes to lose weight and keep it off. First, athletes do not like to follow a programme that markedly restricts the duration and intensity of their training, and second, they do not like to feel hunger when they leave the table after each meal and go to bed each night. On the other hand, many athletes can follow a fat-restricted diet without a deterioration in their training and feeling of well-being. Restricting fat without also restricting calorie intake has been shown to result in weight loss.[35]

Some lay publications advocate a low-fat diet to increase endurance and to improve athletic performance. There is no data to support this view and there is data to refute it.[36]

Some athletes try to restrict caloric intake by sticking their fingers down their throats to induce vomiting. Girls are far more likely than boys to do this. Bulimic athletes usually are brought for medical attention with a chief complaint of a deterioration in athletic performance with weakness and tiredness. They usually deny that they are vomiting. They often appear emaciated and can have severe dental problems. Laboratory tests reveal reduced blood and increased 24-hour urine potassium levels. Vomiting causes loss of large amounts of hydrogen, resulting in a metabolic alkalosis, which prompts the kidneys to try to conserve hydrogen by increasing their output of potassium.

Gaining weight

Some athletes can gain weight just by forcing themselves to eat when they are not hungry. However, much of their weight gain is fat and forcefeeding tends to elevate blood fat levels, which can increase susceptibility to coronary artery disease in later life.

Although most sedentary people store extra fat when they eat more food than they need, many competitive athletes do not. First, vigorous exercise that is required for competitive sports suppresses appetite far more than less intense exercise of shorter duration.[37] Second, a vigorous exercise programme can increase thermogenesis markedly.[38] Furthermore, there is no evidence that eating when not hungry will cause an athlete to grow large muscles.

The only effective way to gain lean body mass is to exercise muscles against progressively greater resistance. To grow large muscles, athletes also need to ingest $1.5g.kg^{-1}.day^{-1}$ of protein.[39] This can be accomplished by most athletes without paying particular attention to protein needs. Physicians and coaches should avoid recommending a high-protein diet. Eating large amounts of protein could limit carbohydrate intake and decrease endurance during workouts and recovery from them.

Table 6.12 4000kcal carbohydrate-rich diet (60% carbohydrate, 15% protein and 25% fat).

Breakfast
1 orange
4 cups of cereal
1 cup of skimmed milk
2 pieces of toast

Snack
Banana

Lunch
Pitta bread
Lettuce and tomato salad
4 ounces tuna fish
Apple
Skimmed milk

Snack
2 slices of bread with peanut butter and jam

Dinner
2 cups mashed potatoes
2 4-ounce breasts of chicken
Large vegetable salad
Apple pie
4 slices of bread

Snack
2 slices of bread
Jam

Table 6.13 A 50kg adolescent needs 75 grams of protein.

1 chicken breast (4 oz)	25 grams protein
4 cups of milk	36
6 ounce can of tuna	48
1 cup dried beans	14
1 cup peanuts	37
3 ounces salmon	17
3 ounces hamburger	25

References

1. Green, H.J. (1991) How important is endogenous muscle glycogen to fatigue in prolonged exercise? *Canad. J. Physiol. Pharmacol.* **69**: 290–297.
2. Felig, P., Cherif, A., Minagawa, A. *et al.* (1982) Hypoglycemia during prolonged exercise in normal men. *New Eng. J. Med.* **306**: 895.
3. Mirkin, G.B. (1983) Food and nutrition for exercise. In: Bove, A.A. and Lowenthal, D.T. (Eds) *Exercise Medicine:*

Physiological Principles and Clinical Applications. Academic Press, New York.

4. Karlsson, J., Nordesjo, L.O. and Saltin, B. (1974) Muscle glycogen utilization during exercise after physical training. *Acta. Physiol. Scand.* **90**: 210.

5. Christensen, E.H. and Hansen, O. (1939) Hypoglykamie, Arbeitsfahigkeit und Ermudung. *Scand. Arch. Physiol.* **81**: 172

6. Astrand, P.O. (1968) Something old and something new - very new. *Nutrition Today* **3(2)**: 9.

7. Mirkin, G.B. (1973) Carbohydrate loading: a dangerous practice. *J. Am. Med. Assoc.* **223**: 1511.

8. Banks, W.J. (1977) Myoglobinuria in marathon runners: possible relationship to carbohydrate and lipid metabolism. *Ann. NY Acad. Sc.* **301**: 942.

9. Sherman, W.M., Costill, D.L., Fink, W., *et al.* (1981) The role of dietary carbohydrates in muscle glycogen resynthesis after strenuous running. *Am. J. Clin. Nutr.* **34**: 1831.

10. Piehl, K. (1974) Time course for refilling of glycogen stores: in human muscle fibres following exercise-induced glycogen depletion. *Acta Physiol. Scand.* **90**: 297.

11. Murray, R., Eddy, D.E., Paul, G.L., Seifert, J.G. and Halaby, G.A. (1991) Physiological responses to glycerol ingestion during exercise. *J. Appl. Physiol.* **71(1)**: 144–149.

12. Hultman, E. and Nilson, L.H. (1971) Liver glycogen in man: effect of different diets on muscular exercise. In: Saltin, B. and Pernow, B. (Eds) *Muscle Metabolism During Exercise*, p. 143. Plenum, New York.

13. Krzentowski, G., Prinay, F., Luyckx, A.S. *et al.* (1984) Effect of physical training on utilization of a glucose load given orally during exercise. *Am. J. Physiol.* **246**: E412.

14. Fielding, R.A., Costill, D.A., Fink, D.S., King, M., Hargreaves, M. and Kovaleski, J.E. (1985) Effect of carbohydrate feeding frequencies and dosage on muscle glycogen use during exercise. *Med. Sci. Sports Exerc.* **17(4)**: 472–476.

15. Kristal-Boneh, E. *et al.* (1988) Improved thermoregulation caused by forced water intake in human desert dwellers. *Eur. J. Appl. Physiol.* **57**: 220–224.

16. Rehrer N, *et al.* (1990) Gastric emptying with repeated drinking during running and bicycling. *Int. J. Sports Med.* **11(3)**: 238–243.

17. *Ibid.*

18. Hargreaves, M., Costill, D.L., Cogan, A. *et al.* (1981) Effects of carbohydrate feeding on muscle glycogen utilization and exercise performance. *Med. Sc. Sports Exerc.* **16**: 219.

19. Costill, D.L., Cote, R., Fink, W.J. *et al.* (1981) Muscle water and electrolyte distribution during prolonged exercise. *Int. J. Sports Med.* **3**: 130.

20. Costill, D.L. and Saltin, B. (1974) Factors limiting gastric emptying during rest and exercise. *J. Appl. Physiol.* **37**: 679.

21. Moore, J.G., Dak, F.L. and Christian, B.S. (1990) Exercise increases solid meal gastric emptying in men. *Dig. Diseases Sc.* **35(4)**: 428–432.

22. Massicotte, D., Peronnet, F., Brisson, G., Bakkouch, K. and Hillaire-Marcel, C. (1989) Oxidation of a glucose polymer during exercise: comparison with glucose and fructose. *J. Appl. Physiol.* **66(1)**: 179–183.

23. Casoni, I., Guglielmini, C., Graziano, L., Reali, M.G., Mazzotta, D. and Abbasciano, V. (1990) Changes of magnesium concentrations in endurance athletes. *Int. J. Sports Med.* **11**: 234–237.

24. Schneider, H., Brouns, F. and Saris, W.H.M. (1991) A rationale for electrolyte replacement during endurance exercise. *Med. Sc. Sports Exerc.* **23(4)**, Suppl.: 768.

25. Rehrer, N.J., Brouns, F., Beckers, E.J., ten Hoor, F. and Saris, W.H.M. (1990) Gastric emptying with repeated drinking during running and bicycling. *Int. J. Sports Med.* **11**: 238–243.

26. Schneider, H., Brouns, F. and Saris, W.H.M. (1991) A rationale for electrolyte replacement during endurance exercise. *Med. Sc. Sports Exerc.* **23(4)**, Suppl.: 768.

27. McArthur, K.E. and Feldman, M. (1989) Gastric acid secretion, gastric release and gastric emptying in humans as affected by liquid meal temperature. *Am. J. Clin. Nutr.* **49**: 51–54.

28. Maughan, R.J. and Lambert, C.P. (1991) Effects of beverage temperature on the appearance of a deuterium tracer in the blood. *Med. Sc. Sports Exerc.* **23(4)**: 584.

29. Zachwieja, J.J., Costill, D.L., Widrick, J.J., Anderson, D.E. and McConell, G.K. (1991) The effects of carbonation on the gastric emptying characteristics of water. *Med. Sc. Sports Exerc.* **23(4)**: S84.

30. Costill, D. *et al.* (1981) The role of dietary carbohydrates in muscle glycogen resynthesis after strenuous running. *Am. J. Clin. Nutr.* **34**: 1831–1836.

31. Ivy, J.L., Katz, A.L., Cutler, C.L., Sherman, W.M. and Coyle, E.F. (1988) Muscle glycogen synthesis after exercise: effect of time on carbohydrate ingestion. *J. Appl. Physiol.* **64**: 1480–1485.

32. Ivy, J.L., Lee, M.C., Brozinick, J.T. and Reed, M.J. (1988) Muscle glycogen storage after different amounts of carbohydrate ingestion. *J. Appl. Physiol.* **65**: 2018–2023.

33. Finch, C.A., Gollnick, P.D., Hlastala, M.P. *et al.* (1979) Lactic acidosis as a result of iron deficiency. *J. Clin. Invest.* **64**: 129.

34. Solomons, N.W. (1986) Competitive interaction of iron and zinc in the diet: consequences for human nutrition. *J. Nutr.* **116**: 926–935.

35. Miller, W.C., Linderman, A.K., Wallace, J. and Niederman, M. (1990) Diet composition, energy intake, and exercise in relation to body fat in men and women. *Am. J. Clin. Nutr.* **52**: 426–430.

36. Kosich, D., Conlee, R., Fischer, A.G. *et al.* (1986) The effects of exercise and a low-fat diet or a moderate-fat diet on selected coronary risk factors. In: Dotson, C. and Humphrey, J. (Eds) *Exercise Physiology: Current Selected Research,* Vol. 2, p. 173. AMS Press, New York.

37. Oscai, L.B. (1973) The role of exercise in weight control. In: Wilmore, J.H. (Ed.) *Exercise and Sports Sciences Reviews,* Vol 1, p. 103. Academic Press, New York.

38. Stern, J.S. and Lowney, P. (1986) Obesity: the role of physical activity. In: Brownell, K.D. and Foreyt, J.P. (Eds) *Handbook of Eating Disorders: Physiology, Psychology, and the Treatment of Obesity, Anorexia, and Bulimia,* p. 145. Basic Books, New York.

39. Paul, F.G. (1989) Dietary protein requirements in physically active individuals. *Sports Med.* **8**: 154.

7. Pre-Participation Sports Examination: Musculo-Skeletal System

George Thabit and Lyle J. Micheli

Childhood athletic participation has dramatically increased over the past twenty years. Children are being introduced to organised sports at increasingly immature stages of physical development. It is not uncommon to find five-year-old 'athletes' participating in dance classes, soccer camps, or martial arts. Pre-participation examination often represents the initial medical contact, and frequently the only medical contact a child will have prior to engaging in potentially injurious activities.

Despite general agreement over the necessity of the pre-participation evaluation, no widely recognised standard examination currently exists. The administrator of a pre-participation evaluation must assess the overall health of the child as well as any conditions which might limit participation or predispose the child athlete to injury.

Under ideal circumstances, the examination is performed by the athlete's primary care physician. A longstanding medical relationship promotes continuity of care and facilitates the safe discussion of important psychosocial issues. In other instances, mass screenings of athletic teams may be performed in an efficient and satisfactory fashion through the coordinated efforts of a team of health care professionals.[2]

A thorough medical history is obtained which includes past hospitalisations, surgery, medication, allergies, tetanus status, family history, menstrual history, and a review of systems. The physical examination should include assessment of height, weight, vision, cardiovascular vital signs, and level of physical maturity. Additionally, evaluation of the skin, chest, lymphatics, abdomen, genitalia, and musculo-skeletal systems must be performed. The physical examination may be specifically focused on problem areas identified by the medical history.

Evaluation of the musculo-skeletal system includes structural integrity and alignment as well as any pre-existing neuro-muscular deficits. Thorough examination of a specific portion of the musculo-skeletal system may be performed should an area of concern be identified in the history and general physical examination. Furthermore, sports-specific musculo-skeletal testing may identify children at risk for injury depending upon the requirements of the activity and the physiological condition of the athlete. Measurement of fitness, strength, and flexibility may reveal specific muscular imbalances or weaknesses. With such knowledge, therapeutic rehabilitative programmes may be instituted prior to the onset of athletic participation.

Sports-specific performance testing reveals an athlete's physical strengths and weaknesses. When testing has been completed the physician may modify the athlete's training programme through exercise prescription. In addition to optimising athletic performance, the data obtained during testing may help to prevent injuries. Although the level of athletic fitness has not yet been proven to decrease the incidence of sports injuries, the presence of specific deficiencies or imbalances in the musculo-skeletal system would seem likely to predispose an individual to injury. The sports-specific testing of fitness includes measurements of body composition, flexibility, strength, endurance, power, speed, agility, balance, and dynamic balance. The performance profile not only helps a child to achieve their athletic potential, but also provides a baseline against which the success of exercise prescription and recovery from injury can be measured.

Information obtained from the medical history, physical examination and any associated sports-specific performance testing allows a personalised athletic profile to be created for the participant. By pairing the profile with the recommendation for participation in competitive sports as published by the American Academy of Pediatrics, a decision regarding clearance for a given sport can be rendered.[1] The decision for clearance is divided into three categories: unrestricted clearance, cleared after notification of either the coach, trainer, or team physician, or clearance deferred until further evaluation by medical specialist.

When properly performed, the pre-participation examination effectively identifies pre-morbid risk factors for the paediatric and adolescent athlete. Medical and social interventions prior to athletic participation may diminish these risks and prevent catastrophic cardiovascular or neurologic events. A yearly evaluation of the growing child is recommended to screen for new health problems, to monitor established conditions and to assess an athlete's preparedness for any given sporting activity.

General appearance examination

Instructions

The athlete stands straight with arms to the side and feet together. General appearance, including the acromioclavicular, sternoclavicular knee and ankle joints, should be symmetrical (**7.1, 7.2**).

7.1 **7.2**

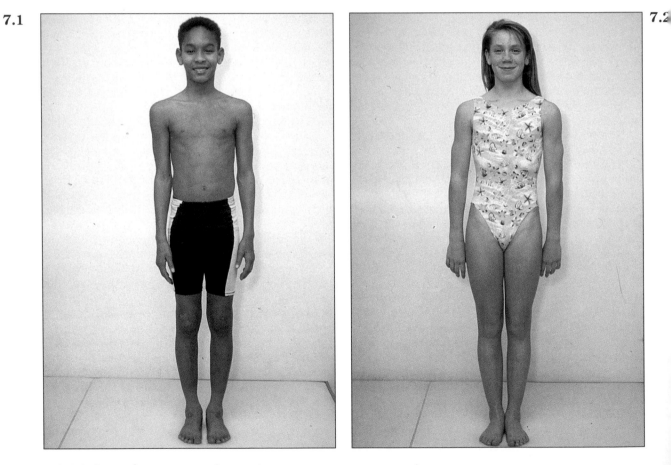

7.1, 7.2 General appearance. Instructions.

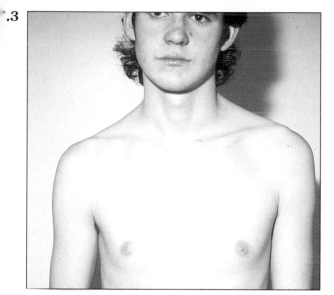

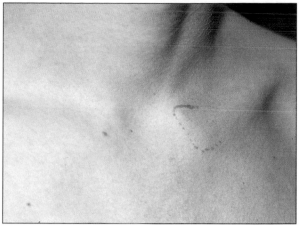

7.3, 7.4 General appearance. Abnormality.

Abnormality

Asymmetry of the examination including chronic swelling or deformity often results from trauma. Chronic dislocation of the sternoclavicular joint typically presents with anterior prominence of the clavicle (**7.3, 7.4**).

Marked femoral internal torsion and compensatory external tibial torsion result in patello-femoral malalignment commonly associated with anterior knee pain and patellar instability (**7.5**).

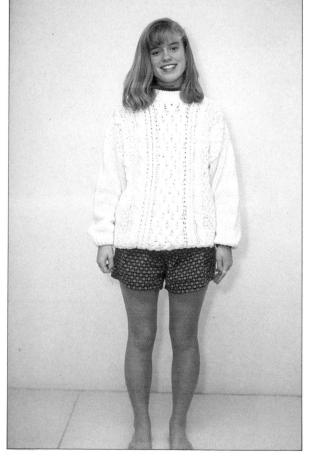

7.5 General appearance. Abnormality.

Cervical spine examination

Instructions

The athlete touches chin to chest (flexion), looks upward (extension), touches ear to shoulder (lateral bending) and looks over each shoulder (lateral rotation). The motion should be symmetrical and pain free (**7.6–7.9**).

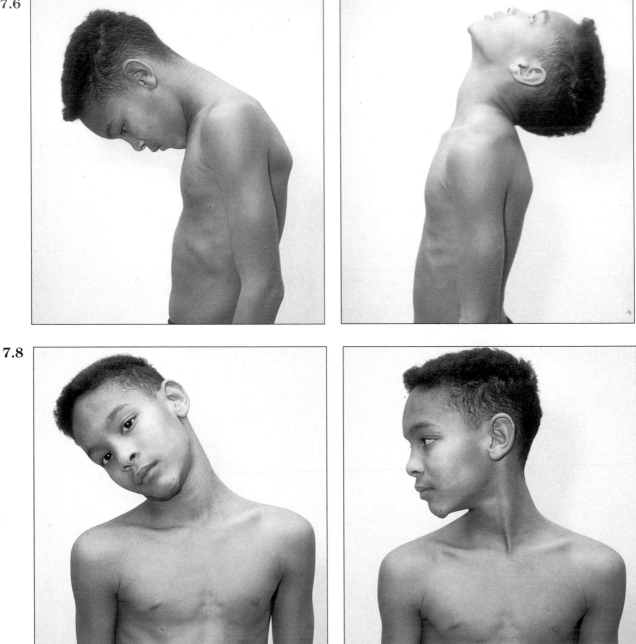

7.6–7.9 Cervical spine examination. Instructions.

Abnormality

Painful or asymmetrical cervical motion often results from traumatic or congenital disorders of the cervical spine. Chronic rotary subluxation of C1–C2 presents as a fixed deformity and a loss of motion (**7.10, 7.11**).

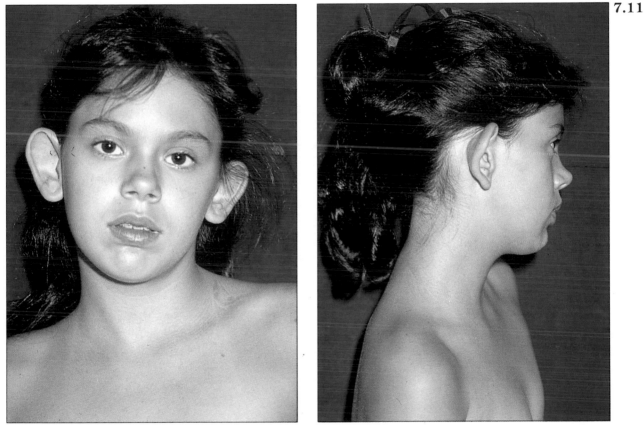

7.10, 7.11 Cervical spine examination. Abnormality.

7.12

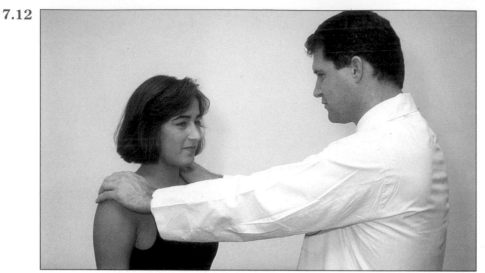

7.12 Neck and shoulder examination. Instructions.

7.13

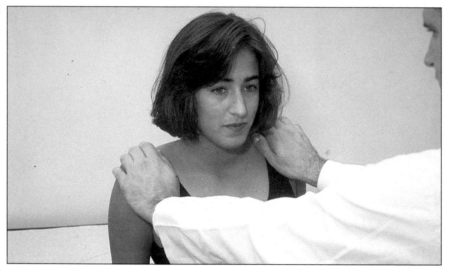

7.13 Neck and shoulder examination. Abnormality.

Neck and shoulder examination

Instructions

Shrug shoulders upward against examiner resistance (**7.12**).

Abnormality

Asymmetry of appearance, motion or strength may indicate cervical or shoulder problems. Asymmetrical shoulder motion is noted in an athlete with a nerve palsy sustained during a skiing accident (**7.13**).

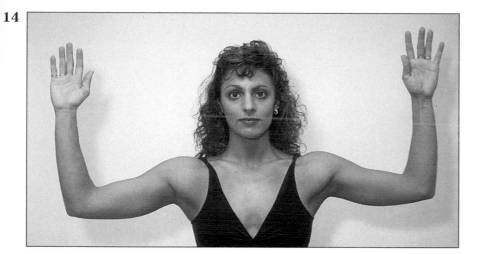

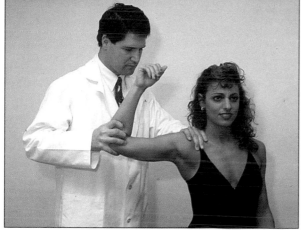

7.14, 7.15 Shoulder examination. Instructions.

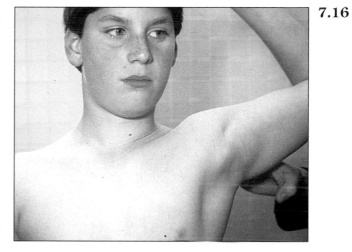

7.16 Shoulder examination. Abnormality.

Shoulder examination

Instructions

Raise arms outward from sides until parallel to the floor. Then flex elbows with hands pointed upwards. The deltoid appearance and strength should be symmetrical. The range of motion of the shoulder should be pain-free and symmetrical (**7.14, 7.15**).

Abnormality

Pain, muscle atrophy, or asymmetrical motion may reflect shoulder instability, impingement or nerve injury. Specific testing of the shoulder will reveal anterior glenohumeral instability as in this athlete with recurrent anterior shoulder dislocations (**7.16**).

7.17

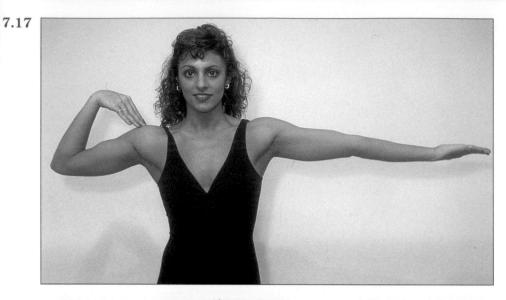

7.17 Elbow examination. Instructions.

7.18

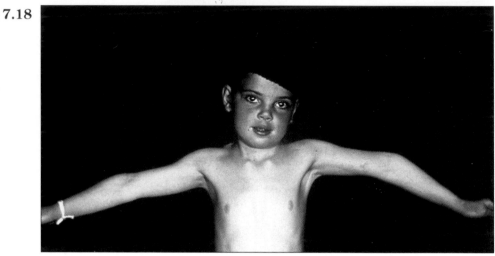

7.18 Elbow examination. Abnormality.

Elbow examination

Instructions

Stand and raise arms out from sides until parallel to the ground. Palms face upward. Alternate elbow flexion and extension. The motion should be symmetrical and pain-free (**7.17**).

Abnormality

Deformity, loss of motion and pain are findings often associated with trauma as seen in this child with a history of a supracondylar fracture of the humerus (**7.18**).

Elbow, forearm, and wrist examination

Instructions

Hold elbows to sides and flex forearms until parallel to the floor. Rotate palms upward and downward in an alternating fashion. The motion should be symmetrical and pain-free (**7.19, 7.20**).

7.19, 7.20 Elbow, forearm and wrist examination. Instructions.

Abnormality

Deformity, loss of motion or pain often accompanies traumatic conditions such as that manifested by a child with a history of an elbow fracture (**7.21**).

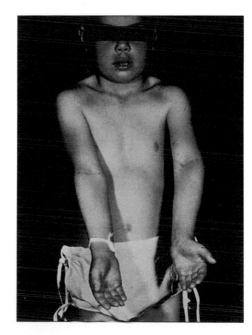

7.21 Elbow, forearm and wrist examination. Abnormality.

Hand examination

Instructions

Clench the fingers into a fist and then spread the fingers wide apart (**7.22, 7.23**).

7.22

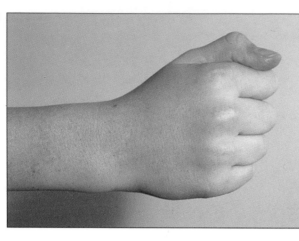

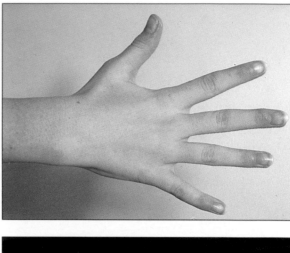

7

7.22, 7.23 Hand examination. Instructions.

Abnormality

Deformity, loss of finger motion or weakness are common post-traumatic findings. Chronic oedema and loss of motion affects this finger subsequent to a proximal interphalangeal joint dislocation (**7.24**).

7.

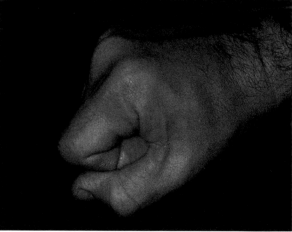

7.24 Hand examination. Abnormality.

Spinal examination

Instructions

The athlete stands straight with back to the examiner and raises arms forward until parallel to the ground. The palms are placed together and the athlete flexes forward to touch their toes. This is repeated with the examiner viewing the athlete from the side. Motion should be pain-free and symmetrical (**7.25–7.28**).

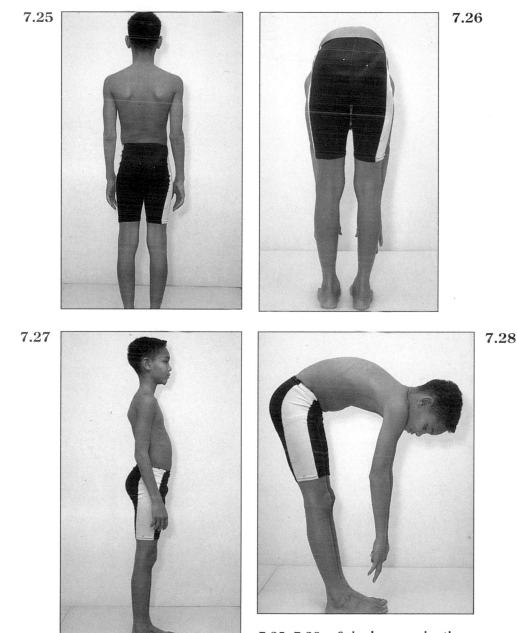

7.25

7.26

7.27

7.28

7.25–7.28 Spinal examination. Instructions.

Abnormality

Pathologic findings include shoulder asymmetry, scapular prominence, pelvic obliquity, cutaneous manifestations of underlying spinal dysraphism and scoliotic and kyphotic deformity. Examples of idiopathic thoracic scoliosis and Scheuermann's kyphosis are presented (**7.29, 7.30**).

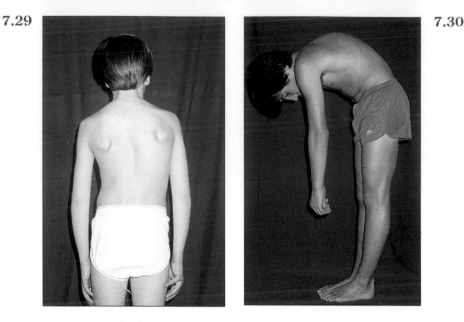

7.29, 7.30 Spinal examination. Abnormality.

Lower extremity examination

Instructions

The athlete squats down on heels, walks four steps in squat position, and then rises to a standing position. This complex activity demonstrates symmetrical lower extremity joint motion and strength. The gait should be pain-free and have equal heel-to-buttock distance. The child should have no difficulty in rising to a standing position (**7.31**).

Abnormality

Hip, knee and ankle problems result in weakness, joint instability or loss of joint motion which preclude a symmetrical duck walk (note heel-to-buttock difference). Specific testing of the affected region will identify the deficiency. Examples of the Lachman and anterior drawer tests which assess competence of the anterior cruciate ligament are presented (**7.32–7.34**).

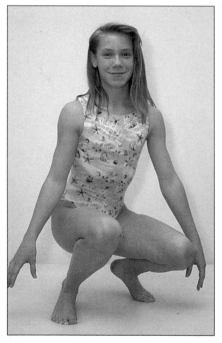

7.31 Lower extremity examination. Instructions.

2

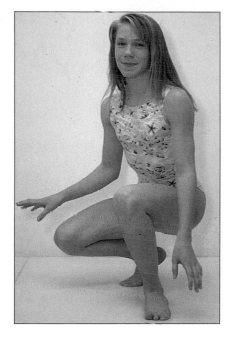

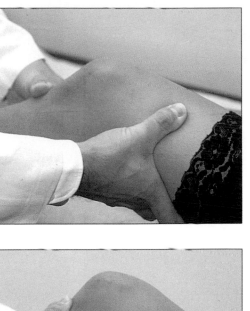

7.33

7.34

7.32–7.34 Lower extremity examination. Abnormality.

Leg and ankle examination

Instructions

The athlete stands straight and then alternately stands on toes and stands on heels. Motion should be pain-free and symmetrical (**7.35–7.37**).

7.35

7.36

7.37

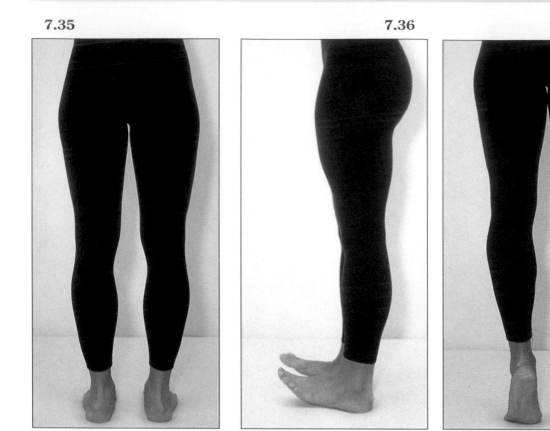

7.35–7.37 Leg and ankle examination. Instructions.

Abnormality

Pathologic findings of the leg examination include muscle atrophy, asymmetry of motion and chronic swelling as seen in this athlete with chronic achilles tendinitis (**7.38**).

References

1. American Academy of Pediatrics Committee on Sports Medicine (1988) Recommendations for participation in competitive sports. *Pediatrics* **81**: 737.
2. Micheli, L.J. and Yost, J.G. (1984) Preparticipation evaluation and first aid for sports. In: Micheli, L.J. (Ed.) *Pediatric and Adolescent Sports Medicine*, pp. 30–48. Little, Brown, Boston.

7.

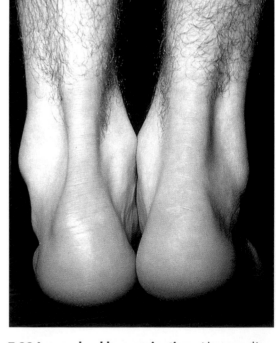

7.38 Leg and ankle examination. Abnormality.

8. Exercise in Children with Chronic Conditions

Nicola Maffulli and Peter Helms

Regular physical exercise is gaining acceptance as a prescription for the prevention, management and rehabilitation of diseases occurring in the paediatric and adolescent age group. Exercise is generally used to increase the physical capabilities of these young patients, but, at times, it can directly influence the evolution of the condition. However, in children with chronic diseases, enhanced physical activity can also be deleterious. For any exercise modality to give a therapeutic effect, it must be performed regularly; an intense, once-in-a-while bout has no place in a long-term, possibly life long, programme. A well structured exercise programme should be implemented, and the children and their carers should collaborate with their physician to adhere to the agreed programme.

This chapter will focus on the physiological and metabolic role of regular exercise in diabetes, asthma and cystic fibrosis, identifying both positive and possible negative effects in these and other conditions.

Cardio-respiratory fitness and its maintenance throughout life is being shown to have important implications for the health of the normal population, and may modify or reduce the natural decline in organ function that occurs with ageing. The effects of ageing on the decline in lung function are well known, as are the deleterious effects of exposure to cigarette smoking (**8.1**). The effects of disease can be seen as summative or as an earlier and accelerated ageing process. Some of these effects may be reduced by simple health measures such as an increase in activity and regular exercise. The usual decline in cardio-respiratory fitness seen in adolescent girls can, for example, be reversed with regular sustained exercise (**8.2, 8.3**).

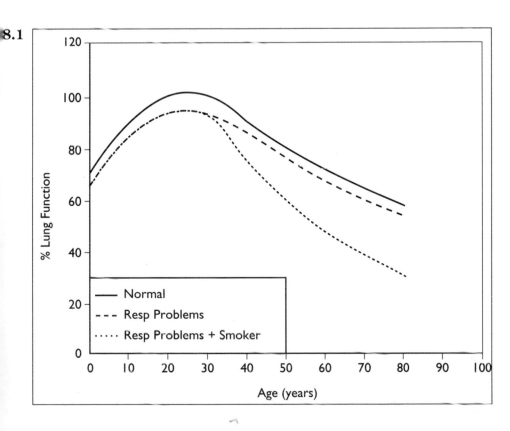

8.1 Effects of maturation and ageing on lung function after taking growth in body size into account. Note the later effects of respiratory problems in early childhood and the additional deleterious effects of smoking.

8.2

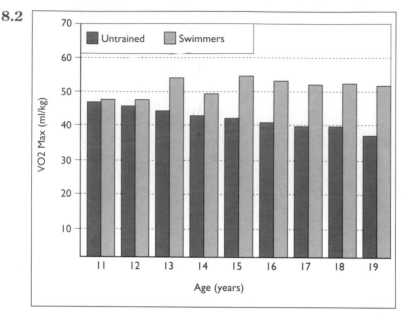

8.2 Development of cardio-respiratory fitness as assessed by maximal oxygen uptake ($\dot{V}O_2$max) during exercise in sedentary and elite swimmers. Note the decline in sedentary girls which is reversed in swimmers.

8.3 Assessment of cardio-respiratory fitness by maximal oxygen uptake ($\dot{V}O_2$max) on a treadmill.

8.3

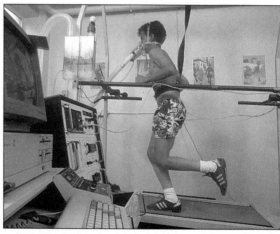

Asthma

The normal sensation of breathlessness during exercise has great significance for asthma sufferers because this is likely to remind the child of the unpleasant features of attacks of the disease. This may lead to exercise avoidance and a cycle of inactivity and physical deterioration. Indeed, several studies have shown the relative 'unfitness' of asthmatic children and adolescents.

In addition, the very act of exercise is likely to provoke an episode of wheezing. This is particularly so in asthmatic children in whom over 80% will respond in this way. The underlying mechanism appears to be due to airway cooling and evaporative water loss from the airway epithelium. There is also good evidence that intensity of exercise is another important factor. Whatever the underlying cause, much of this abnormal response can be blocked by prior administration with beta$_2$ stimulants and/or chromoglycate.

Moderate levels of exercise can therefore be safely undertaken by almost any affected individual, and more intense and sustained levels need not be avoided, as evidenced by the number of world class athletes who suffer from asthma. Training significantly increases aerobic power in asthmatic children (**8.4**), and may even reduce their need for

8.4

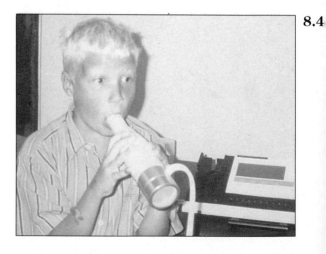

8.4 Assessment of lung function in a child with asthma.

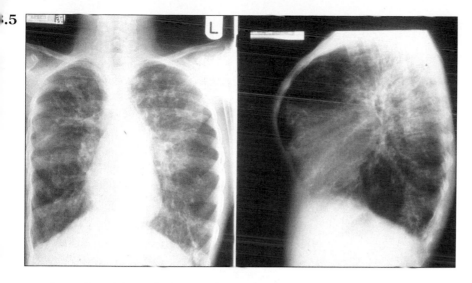

8.5 Frontal and lateral chest radiograph in a severely affected individual with cystic fibrosis. Note the marked hyperinflation and areas of atelectasis, and cystic dilation due to bronchiectasis.

anti-asthmatic drugs, the frequency of attacks and hospitalisation rate. Swimming is the sport universally recommended for asthmatics, but, with proper warming-up exercises, use of beta-agonists by inhalation and reduction of dry cold air inspiration, any sport can be practised. Swimming without an adequate warm-up may exert potentially dangerous effects due the the diving reflex, which produces bronchoconstriction secondary to enhanced parasympathetic drive.

Cystic fibrosis

Cystic fibrosis is the most common genetically-inherited disease affecting Caucasian population, with a live birth incidence of approximately of 1 in 2000. With improved medical management, life expectancy has increased dramatically since the disease was first described over five decades ago. The vast majority of affected children will now survive into adult life. Pulmonary disease remains the greatest threat to life and health, and, although the patterns of symptoms are different from those in children with asthma (**8.5**), a similar reluctance to undertake regular exercise is often found. However, when exercise programmes have been developed, often in combination with physio-therapy, they have proved safe and popular.

Greater respiratory muscle endurance, improved lung function and greater airway mucus clearance have been described following a period of regular exercise in children with this disease, and there is some evidence that the progressive decline in respiratory status can be slowed in children undertaking regular sustained activity. However, the physician should be aware of the risks of profuse exercise-induced sweating, resulting in large, and difficult to quantify, losses of salt (the basic defect involves increased loss of chloride and sodium in sweat). There is also the possibility of arterial blood desaturation at high intensity of effort, and, with the increased popularity of skiing holidays, this can be exacerbated by altitude. Patients should be educated not to over-exert themselves, to drink plenty of fluids and to replace salt loss.

Diabetes

It is not possible to unequivocally answer the question whether appropriate forms of sporting activities prolong life expectancy and decrease the complication rate in this condition. Some retro-spective studies have shown a reduced prevalence of microangiopathy in young patients undergoing a regime of regular physical activity, and some short-term prospective studies have shown that physical exercise decreases the risk of developing macro-angiopathy in diabetic children.

It is still relatively common to hear that parents, teachers and doctors tend to limit a diabetic child, possibly because they are not fully aware of the problem, and because of unjustified fears.

At the beginning of any physical activity, muscle glycogen is the main energy source. However, if activity is sustained, plasma glucose and free fatty acids (FFA), adopt greater significance. The increased peripheral carbohydrate needs during muscle exercise are met by a higher rate of hepatic glucose production through glycogenolysis, and, during very prolonged exercise, by neoglucogenesis.

Muscle glucose utilisation is dependent on several factors. Among these, of greater importance for the young diabetic, are:

- Insulin, which is a regulating factor in glucose uptake.
- An increased blood flow, which favours glucose availability to muscles.
- An enhanced sensitivity of insulin receptors, which increases peripheral glucose utilisation.
- Local hypoxia, that could be a stimulus for glucose uptake.

Regular physical activity exerts a beneficial effect on the clinical picture of diabetes, favouring glucose, FFA and ketone bodies utilisation, better capillarisation, and improving blood flow and peripheral exchanges.

In normal individuals, the risk of exercise-associated hypoglycaemia is low, as plasma glucose tends to remain constant. In the case of a relative insulin deficiency, increased liver glucose production is not balanced by increased peripheral uptake, and even moderate exercise may sometimes induce hyperglycaemia, possibly leading to severe ketoacidosis.

In exercising diabetic patients with good metabolic control, plasma glucose will be reduced, and there will be a less pronounced increase of ketone bodies, FFA, lactate and pyruvate, cortisol, glucagon and catecholamines. In this situation, hypoglycaemia is always a potential problem, and supplemental glucose should always be available.

Some rheological characteristics of the blood, especially in diabetics with poor metabolic control, can impair oxygen delivery to the tissues.

After exercise, both in the fasting and post-prandial state, there is an increase in the binding of insulin to erythrocytes, as a consequence of the greater number of receptors present in individuals with diabetes. These receptors show no relation with the plasma levels of insulin, glucagon, FFA, ketone bodies and lactate.

During more prolonged exercise, the decrease in muscle glycogen stimulates glycogen synthase and plasma glucose utilisation by the muscles.

Although few studies have been performed on diabetics, there is no reason why regular physical exercise should not produce raised serum HDL cholesterol and 2-3 DPG, and decreased LDL cholesterol and triglycerides, as shown in healthy subjects.

In a non-conditioned diabetic patient, a sudden, heavy effort represents a highly stressful situation, with consequent risk of metabolic control. For example, a sudden increase of plasma glucagon, the greater sensitivity to it by a diabetic patient, and the tendency to eat when hypoglycaemia occurs, may all lead to hyperglycaemia. Moreover, the development of microalbuminuria in previously non-albuminuric patients raises some concerns about the safety of regular sustained exercise in diabetes.

Microalbuminuria is a normal feature of exercise in healthy subjects, but, in diabetics, very strenuous exercise may be harmful, as an increased glomerular protein flow may exacerbate existing renal angiopathy and local tissue damage. A less intense and regular form of physical exercise is not associated with proteinuria. In the presence of diabetic microangiopathy, heavy exercise is probably contra-indicated.

A decreased ability to vasodilate, together with increased transglomerular protein loss and redistribution of blood flow towards the working muscles, can prolong the negative effects of hypoxia. Diabetic patients with nephropathy are at risk of cerebral ischaemia, and the onset of hypertension can worsen an early retinopathy, again a potent reason for caution in the prescription of exercise in severely affected individuals.

From a practical viewpoint, a young diabetic patient should:

- Increase his/her caloric intake during intense, prolonged exercise.
- He/she should decrease insulin administration if, after a test period of exercise, hypoglycaemia is present. This should be achieved by adjusting the dose of rapid-acting insulin rather than changing medium-/long-acting dosage.

Well controlled young diabetic patients should take part in school and recreational sports, although some care should be taken in high intensity and sustained exercise, particularly in those with advanced disease.

There is a psychological benefit to be had from regular physical activity. Anxiety is reduced and, above all, diabetic children may feel more equal to their healthy peers. In this regard, the role of the doctor must be as an educator, and his/her aim should be to lead the diabetic child to a full and independent lifestyle.

Arterial hypertension

Although the effects of chronic exercise programmes are well established in hypertensive adults, similar benefits have not been irrevocably proven in hypertensive adolescents. Violent exercise may result in very high systolic and diastolic blood pressure, and thus prolonged aerobic exercise should be encouraged. However, a long-term programme of weight training in hypertensive 14- to 18-year-old adolescents has shown a mild decrease in resting blood pressure. Recently, the 16th Bethesda Conference on Cardiovascular Abnormalities in Athletes suggested free sports participation to hypertensive adolescents without secondary organ damage and whose diastolic blood pressure did not exceed 115mmHg. It is probably wise to avoid contact sports and the attendant risk of acute tissue injuries, particularly head injuries.

Myopathies

Exercise results in exceptionally high levels of serum intra-muscular enzymes, such as creatine kinase and myoglobin, implying muscle fibre damage, and it is generally thought that dystrophic changes could be accelerated during exercise. However, very little damage is generally found in post-mortem studies of respiratory muscles. In animal models, it has been shown that high intensity training accelerates the degenerative myopathic process, whilst no significant damage was found following aerobic training. Furthermore, there is no clear relationship between the elevation of serum intra-muscular enzymes and the extent of histologically demonstrable muscle damage.

There is therefore no definite proof that exercise accelerates the course of the disease, and probably a mild to moderate intensity exercise programme should be implemented in young children well before they develop muscle imbalance. Maintenance of continuous movement following surgical management of the contractures that inevitably develop is likely to speed recovery. Very short perods of immobilisation are recommended, and walking and active physiotherapy are encouraged within 24 hours of surgery.

Conclusions

A programme of regular exercise can be beneficial to the medical and psychological management of chronic disease in children and adolescents. The effects of isolated and intense exercise are detrimental, and should be discouraged. A well-planned training and exercise programme appropriate for the individual and medical problem can enhance the quality of life in children with chronic illness (**8.6**).

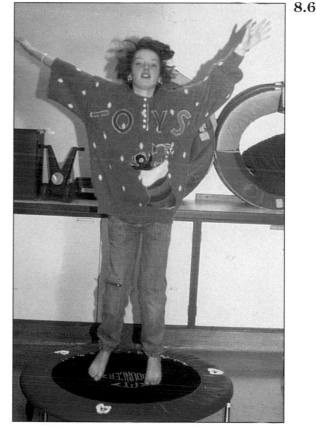

8.6

8.6 Exercise as part of a chest physiotherapy regime using a portable trampoline.

Suggested reading

Anon. (1989) Exercise training, fitness and asthma. *Lancet* 763–764.

Cerny, F.J. and Armitage, L.M. (1989) Exercise and cystic fibrosis. *Pediatr. Exerc. Sci.* **1**: 116–126.

Fowler, W.M. and Taylor, M. (1982) Rehabilitation management of muscular dystrophy and related disorders. The role of exercise. *Arch. Phys. Med. Rehabil.* **63**: 319–321.

Kemmer, F.W. and Berger, M. (1983) Exercise and diabetes mellitus: physical activity as part of daily life and its role in treatment of diabetic patients. *Int. J. Sports Med.* **4**: 77.

Maffulli, N. (1992) Sports activity in diabetic children. *Sports Med. and Soft Tissue Trauma* **4**: 4–5.

Marliss, E.B. and Zinman, B. (1981) Exercise and diabetes. *Diabetologia* **21**: 237.

McMillan, D.E. (1979) Exercise and diabetic microangiopathy. *Diabetes* **28**: 103.

Rowland, T.N. (1990) *Exercise and Children's Health.* Human Kinetics Publisher, Champaign, Ill.

Schartzstein, R.M. (1992) Asthma: to run or not to run? *Am. Rev. Respir. Dis.* **145**: 739–740.

Speechly, D.N.E., Rimmer, S.J. and Hodson, M.E. (1992) Exacerbation of cystic fibrosis after holidays at high altitude. A cautionary tale. *Respir. Med.* **86**: 55–56.

Stanghelle, J.R., Skyberg, D. and Hannaes, O.C. (1992) Eight-year follow-up of pulmonary function and oxygen uptake during exercise in 16-year-old males with cystic fibrosis. *Acta Paediatr.* **81**: 527–531.

9. Stress and the Young Athlete: A Psychological Perspective

Ze'ev Levita and Nicola Maffulli

What is stress

Stress is a complicated concept, as it implies different things to different people. However, three conceptually different definitions emerge from stress research literature.

Stress as a response

In this instance, stress is conceived as a physiological response to any type of demand made upon the body. Stress, therefore is the accumulation of all the (mainly) somatic physiological responses. These bodily responses have a defensive purpose, and their main function is to resist and cope with the unusual demands made upon the body.

Stress in children involved in sport, therefore, consists of their physiological response to the unusual, and additional, physical demands made by the requirements of training and competition. Other demands can also be considered, such as the changes in those children's lifestyles as imposed by training requirements.

Many physiological, or stress, responses have been investigated. They include pulse rate, blood pressure, erythrocyte sedimentation rate, protein-bound iodine, serum iron, serum cholesterol, high- and low-density lipoproteins, serum cortisol, thyroid hormones, serum glucose, serum uric acid, catecholamine excretion and so forth.

Stress as a stimulus

From this point of view, stress is defined and measured in terms of the demands made on the organism. These demands range from straightforward physical stimuli like noise, light, heat and so forth, through demands like workload, pace of work and complexity of demand, to even more complicated variables that include socio-psychological components like isolation and confinement, group pressure, frustration, crowding and role conflict.

Children in sport confront many different stressful stimuli and situations, from the physical demands directly related to their sporting endeavour to their environmental training conditions (e.g. size, illumination and ventilation of their gymnasium) through more complex factors. Children who engage in sport are often isolated from their sedentary peers, their parents and siblings. They are subject to group pressure and pressure of expectations by parents, trainers and sponsors, including those imposed by their own hopes and ambitions.

Training and competitions expose them to various frustrations related to failure to meet standards, deterioration in performance due to tiredness/exhaustion, emotional/mental factors, injury and social circumstances. It is reasonable to assume that, on many occasions, the demands made on children are conflicting (e.g. high grades in their school exams, and being selected to first junior team/squad).

Transactional definitions of stress

The conviction behind this type of definition is that stress is best understood in terms of transaction between demands made on the organism and the resources available to the organism to meet those demands. More sophisticated models of stress refer to it in terms of P/E fit, i.e. fit between the Person and the Environment.

The environment exerts certain demands but also supplies satisfaction for particular needs. The person has certain needs that have to be satisfied and has given resources (abilities, etc.) to meet the various environmental demands. The stress is created when there is a disparity (lack of fit) either between demands and resources, or between the needs and satisfactions which the environment can supply.

One of the interesting logical consequences of this type of model is that one can suffer from stress when one's resources exceed demand (e.g. overqualified for a certain level of competition), or when one's needs are less (or different) than the satisfactions offered by the environment.

The young athlete's situation viewed from this frame of reference is quite unique. Most children and young people who take up sport seriously are blessed with talent and physical attributes. Here lie two types of trap. One: as they are talented, having high resources, the demands made on them are high. The danger here is that they may be too high. Equally, when one has to consider that resources also mean mental and emotional resources, these in a young athlete do not necessarily equal the physical resources. They are children or adolescents with the mental and emotional maturity that this implies.

The other trap is that the demands made on them can be lower than their resources. This can also result in stress. It is not uncommon to meet bored, unhappy young people who are not being challenged in proportion to their aptitudes and abilities. In contrast to popular belief, lack of demand does not make a person happy and satisfied, especially if the person is very capable. Children's and young people's needs should also be taken into account. Needs that are relevant to children and young people are, in many circumstances, ignored in a sport-competitive environment that emphasises needs and motives based on adult value-systems. It can happen that a young child's needs for security, warmth, protection and unconditional love are not met in an environment that promotes toughness, task-orientated achievement, motivation, self-reliance and maturity.

Although aggressive needs are argued to be satisfied through sports activities, it is doubtful that they are satisfied in the same sense as in a regular environment. Sport has been classically regarded as a sublimation of aggressive urges. Nevertheless, it should be pointed out that the sport environment emphasises self-discipline and control, i.e. 'playing by the rules', which does not always allow for the satisfaction of aggressive needs otherwise met by young people outside the structured 'professional' sport environment.

The Person-Environment fit (P/E fit) cannot be measured in objective terms only. We have to bear in mind that stress, ultimately, is a personal matter. This means that what really matters is the person's perception of all the P/E fit elements. These include his/her private perception of environmental demands and supplies, and his/her personal perception of his/her own abilities and needs. Stress can be therefore defined as 'subjective perception of P/E fit'.

This implies that personal perception will not necessarily agree with 'objective' measurement of P/E fit by others. For example, a young person can be overwhelmed by his/her personal estimation of other competitors' ability (part of the E) and undervalue his/her own ability (P), creating a subjective P/E misfit. This may result in stress, although, objectively, there is no P/E misfit because the child's abilities are on a par with, or even higher, than those of the competitors.

It is important to remember that, when children and young persons are involved, one cannot always expect them to be good realistic estimators of P/E fit. Indeed, one cannot always expect that from adults.

Adolescents provide a good example of this. With their typical fluctuation between need for support, reassurance and protection on the one hand, and self-assertion and independence on the other, it is very difficult to meet those conflicting expectations in a way which will be perceived by the adolescent as fitting his/her needs. When subjective perception is taken into account, within the context of the emotional and social development of children and young persons, it is easy to see the many possible sources of stress for young athletes.

This may also explain the many instances where a young person is extremely stressed although others cannot perceive any reason for this. To put things into the right perspective, one has to note that mature athletes are not necessarily immune to stress as they also face many situations of, objectively or subjectively, perceived P/E misfit.

The sources of stress for children and young athletes are unique and very much related to their specific emotional, social and cognitive development.

Those issues have to be taken into account if children's and young athletes' stress is to be understood before proper preventive intervention measures are taken.

The research in the field of stress has mainly focused on mature athletes. Investigation of adult and some junior samples indicates that the participants themselves identify the following areas as main sources of stress: fear of failure, making mistakes, concern about expectations of others, poor preparatory training, physical state, the media and unforseen events. All those elements could be accomodated into the P/E fit model, either as need/satisfaction or as resources/demands objective or subjective misfit.

Actual injury is an obvious source of stress. Inability to perform as a result of injury can be conceptualised as needs/satisfaction misfit, and commencing training/competition after injury as abilities/demands misfit.

Generalisation of those findings in children should be cautious. In the same way as children's needs and resources are different from adults, as are their perceptions and interpretations of external and internal environment, so are their specific areas or sources of stress. This should be more closely investigated, but the best approach for the parents, carers and coaches/trainers would probably be to be aware of the possible sources of P/E misfit and the children's and young adults' own private perception and interpretation of the situation. Better understanding of the young athlete's personal interpretation of his/her situation will allow better understanding of the relevant sources of stress, thus providing opportunity for proper prevention, preparation and intervention.

One final word of caution. It is not presently proven that stress is necessarily an evil. On the contrary, some evidence shows that stress, of certain quality and quantity, can act as a positive incentive.

Stress. So what?

Many would argue that stress is a fact of life. Stress cannot be reduced, therefore it has to be lived with, either as a necessary evil, or a beneficial evil. Nevertheless, in sport, stress is a relevant issue, as it is evidently related to level of performance and propensity for injury.

The most important factor is the child or young person. People are not passive respondents to stimuli. People are pro-active and reflective. This means that they reflect upon, interpret and ascribe meaning to things that happen to them, including their own perception of P/E fit or misfit. Therefore, it is reasonable to assume that, if a child defines a certain demand/resource or need/satisfaction misfit as challenging or as threatening, it will result in different performance outcomes.

In relation to behaviour in general, and sport performance in particular, stress cannot be seriously discussed without taking into account coping processes. Therefore, not only the level of stress as such, but also the coping processes the person uses in order to withstand and/or overcome stress, are important. Evidence exists to indicate that people who use emotionally-oriented coping cope less well with stress than people who use problem-oriented coping.

The coping strategies young people use depends very much on their previous experiences, emotional and social maturity. They also depend on their interpretation of the situation and the personal meaning of the situation.

Coping efforts, on a higher, cognitive level, may change the meaning of a situation, including internally-perceived P/E fit/misfit, in such a way that it renders the whole situation less stressful. This type of higher-level cognitive coping (or cognitive control of stress) very much depends on cognitive maturity and cognitive skills. Nevertheless, there is no reason why children and young persons should not be encouraged to learn and to use these skills .

Injury is the proverbial nemesis of sport. Most of the factors contributing to sport injury are physical or physiological, such as poor equipment, poor field conditions, weather, nature of sport, training status, over-training, and so forth. Nevertheless, psychological factors, including those related to stress, cannot be overlooked. Although there is a lack of experimental evidence regarding the relation between stress and injury in children, such evidence in adults indicates that stress is a contributing factor in injury, even if not the most direct and important one. For example, people who suffered from more stressful life-events were found to suffer more injuries.

Personality factors also seem to be involved. For example, tough-minded people are less likely to receive injuries, while people with high trait-anxiety run a greater risk of injury. Coping skills and social support moderate the effects of stress on injury. People with poor coping skills and low social support are particularly vulnerable to stress-related injury.

Research on stress related injuries is focused on adult athletes, and data on children is mostly of a circumstantial nature. As a consequence, generalisation to children should be made cautiously. Nevertheless, many coaches who work with children admit that some children and young adults are more injury-prone than others, and that accidents seem to happen to those children more frequently involved in stressful situations.

Suggested reading

Andersen, M.B. and Williams, J.M. (1988) A model of stress and athletic injury: prediction and prevention. *J. Sport Exerc. Psychol.* **10**: 294–306.

Cox, T. (1978) *Stress*. University Park Press, Baltimore.

Hardy, L. (1992) Psychological stress, performance and injury in sport. *Br. Med. Bull.* **48**: 615–629.

Jones, J.G. and Hardy, L. (1990) *Stress and Performance in Sport*. John Wiley & Sons, New York.

Roberts, C.G. and Darren, C. (1992) Children in sport. *Sport Sci. Rev.* **1**: 46–64.

Rowley, S. and Maffulli, N. (1990) Gli effetti psicologici dell'allenamento intenso in giovani atleti. *Medicina dello Sport* **43**: 49–53.

10. Gynaecological Issues for the Young Female Athlete

Pasquale Patrizio, C. Terence Lee and Nicola Maffulli

In the past few years, an increasing number of women have undertaken full-time competitive sports training. Many of them start their training prior to puberty, and continue their rigorous activity throughout the childbearing years. As a result, gynaecologists are now confronted with new issues related to women and exercise.

The aim of this chapter is to address some of the problems a young female athlete may encounter during her career.

Oral contraceptives

Although oral contraceptives (OCPs) have not been shown to significantly alter sporting performance, many athletic women are concerned about their potential side effects, such as weight gain, water retention, breakthrough bleeding and mood changes. There is also concern about potentially serious complications such as thromboembolic disease, cancer and cardiovascular risks.

However, the benefits of OCPs actually surpass their risks (**10.1**). Besides being an excellent method of contraception, they can be beneficial in decreasing the amount of menstrual bleeding and the degree of cramping, as well as lowering the incidence of ovarian cancer, endometrial cancer and benign ovarian cysts (**10.2**).

OCPs can also be used to regulate the timing of menstrual cycles, so as not to coincide with important athletic events. However, routine use of this practice is not recommended.

Standard OCPs do not show up in routine anti-doping screening.

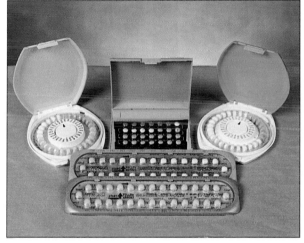

10.1 Oral contraceptives have several non-contraceptive benefits.

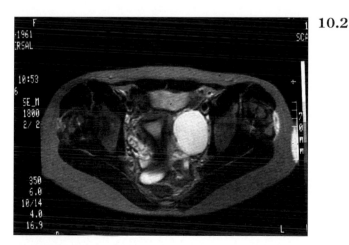

10.2 MRI of ovarian cyst. Oral contraceptive use may help suppress functional cysts.

Breast injuries

High-impact sport may cause some degree of trauma to the breasts when they strike against the chest wall. Common problems include nipple irritation as a result of rubbing against non-supportive brasserie or coarse clothing during physical activity. This sometimes becomes severe enough to cause bleeding. Any bleeding from the nipples should be evaluated by a specialist to rule out more serious causes, such as certain tumours.

Sports involving projectiles and chest-wall impact may result in breast haematomas (**10.3**). These involve bleeding from deep veins and usually resolve spontaneously within 2–3 weeks.

Athletes should wear specially-fitted bras made from non-abraslve, inelastic material so as to provide adequate support.

Some athletes and dancers with large breasts have benefitted from surgery to reduce breast size (**10.4, 10.5**). Athletes wishing to obtain further advice regarding this option, or those considering breast augmentation (**10.6, 10.7**), should consult a certified plastic surgeon.

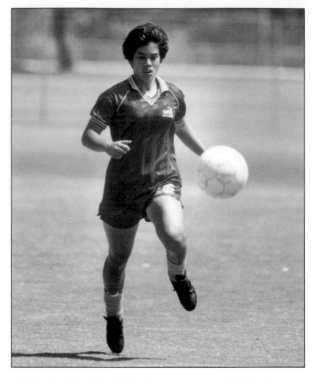

10.3 Projectile injuries may result in breast haematomas.

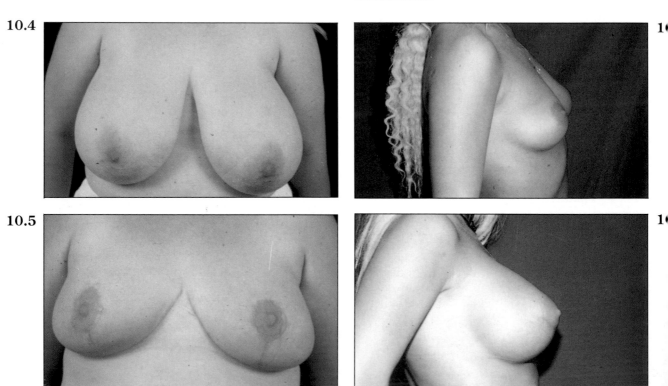

10.4, 10.5 Breast reduction may help athletic performance in some women.

10.6, 10.7 Breast augmentation, although not absolutely contraindicated, is not recommended in serious athletes.

Vulvar haematoma

Vulvar haematomas in the majority of cases result from direct trauma to the genital organs during activities such as bicycle riding, gymnastics, horse riding or water skiing (**10.8**). Conservative treatment with ice packs and pain medications is usually successful. If the haematoma does not resolve, it may need to be drained surgically to isolate and stop the bleeding vessel.

Amenorrhoea

Maintainance of regular menstruation is a complex process involving the central nervous system, the hypothalamus, the pituitary gland, the ovaries and the uterus.

Endurance athletes show a greater prevalence of menstrual problems than the general population (**10.9**, **10.10**). These problems include primary amenorrhoea (a delay in the onset of the first menstrual period) and secondary amenorrhoea (a cessation of menses in girls who have already started menstruating).

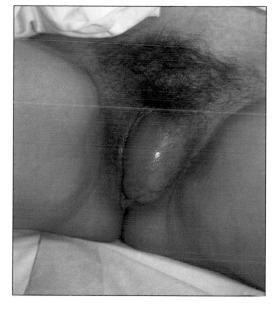

10.8 Vulvar haematoma may result from gymnastics, bicycle riding or horseback riding.

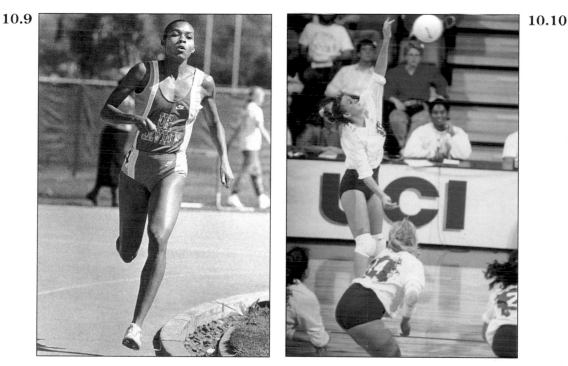

10.9

10.10

10.9, 10.10 Amenorrhoea can occur in long-distance runners and other endurance athletes, gymnasts and ballet dancers.

Many theories have been proposed to explain why athletes are more susceptible to these menstrual irregularities. The most commonly cited one states that low levels of body fat are instrumental in causing menstrual dysfunctions. However, most of the studies supporting this claim have major design errors.

According to a more scientifically-substantiated belief, the mechanism would be multifactorial, with exercise itself having transient effects on the hypothalamic-pituitary-ovarian axis. These effects are also influenced by nutritional and psychological factors.

Despite all this, an athlete who develops amenorrhoea should be treated just as a non-athlete, in the sense that a careful evaluation should be performed to rule out hyperandrogenism, thyroid disorders, prolactin disorders and premature ovarian failure. Only then can the amenorrhoea be attributed to her exercise status.

The main reason for intervention if the patient becomes amenorrhoeic is the prevention of bone loss. Hypo-oestrogenism can lead to decreased bone density, leading to osteoporosis. Treatment is by oestrogen supplementation, for which OCPs can be used, and/or by a change in training habits.

Luteal phase disturbance

Some athletes, despite normal menses, can still have hormonal disturbances. These include delayed puberty and luteal phase defects. The luteal phase (the time between ovulation and menses), normally lasts between 10 and 12 days. It has been demonstrated by recording basal body temperatures, and serum progesterone assays that luteal phase disruption can reverse when the intensity of training is reduced.

Luteal phase defects and amenorrhoea should not be allowed to continue untreated.

Candida infections

Candida, or yeast, is found in 25% of women as part of the normal vaginal environment. Though many women are asymptomatic, some will complain of itching and burning. A large number of contributing factors to the exacerbation of candida infections have been proposed, including diabetes, immuno-suppression and tight-fitting clothing. It is not a sexually-transmitted disease, and treatment can be instituted with clotrimazole. However, any new vaginal discharge should first be evaluated by a physician to rule out other serious infections.

Toxic shock syndrome

Toxic shock syndrome is a systemic infection caused by bacterial toxins, with the majority of cases occurring in young healthy women who use tampons. Patients will complain of a sudden onset of fever, headache, vomiting, body aches and a sunburn-like rash. Immediate medical therapy with antibiotics and intravenous hydration should be instituted once the diagnosis has been made.

Recurrence rates are high, so women who have suffered from this condition should not use tampons, or at least should change them every 4–6 hours and to avoid using them while sleeping.

Acknowledgements

The photos were courtesy of Garth Fisher MD and John Williams MD, Aesthetica Surgical Center, 5757 Wilshire Boulevard, Los Angeles, CA 90036, USA, and of UC-Irvlne Women's Athletics Department.

Suggested reading

Hale, R.W. (1991) *Caring for the Exercising Woman.* Elsevier, New York.

Shangold, M. and Mirkin, G. (1985) *The Complete Sports Medicine Book for Women.* Simon and Schuster.

Shangold, M. and Mirkin, G. (1988) *Women and Exercise: Physiology and Sports Medicine.* F.A. Davis, Philadelphia.

Montagnani, C.F., Arena, B. and Maffulli, N. (1992) Estradiol and progesterone during exercise in healthy untrained women. *Med. Sci. Sports Exer.* **24**: 764–768.

Maffulli,N. and Arena, B. (1993) Menstrual cycle and performance in female athletes. *Obst. Gynaecol. Today* **4**: 6–9.

11 Muscle Strength and Training in Children

D.A. Jones and M.E. Mills

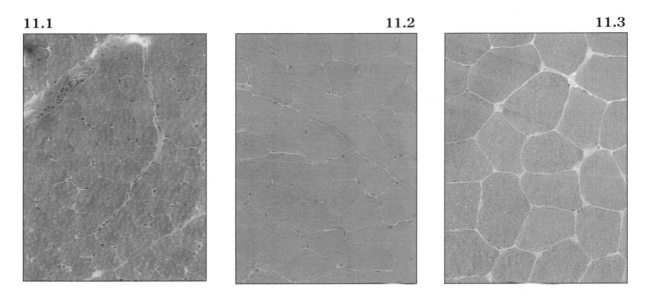

11.1–11.3 Transverse sections of muscle biopsies taken from the quadriceps muscles of a 5-year-old boy (**11.1**), a 12-year-old boy (**11.2**) and a 30-year-old man (**11.3**). All sections are stained with Trichrome and photographed at the same magnification. Note the increasing size of the fibres with increasing age, size and strength of the muscles.

Growth and development of skeletal muscle

Skeletal muscle, unlike the majority of tissue, is composed of multinucleate cells, or fibres, which are formed by the fusion of myoblasts at a comparatively early stage in gestation. Closely associated with the fibres are small undifferentiated satellite cells. Muscle growth involves the division of these mononuclear cells and the fusion of one of the daughter nuclei with the muscle fibre, thereby increasing the nuclear mass and ultimately the size of the muscle fibre. Growth is thought to proceed by an increase in size of existing muscle fibres while the number of fibres remains constant.

Skeletal muscles are fully formed and the fibres differentiated into the characteristic fast and slow types at, or soon after, birth. The fibres are, however, small and over the next 12 to 20 years they grow in diameter and length to reach adult size (**11.1–11.3**). There is a steady and similar increase in strength of boys and girls up to the age of puberty when there is a rapid increase in strength of boys which is not matched by changes in girls (**11.4, 11.5**). The difference in strength between young adult men and women is almost entirely a question of muscle fibre size. Figures **11.6, 11.7** illustrate the difference in fibre size between an adult man and woman. Estimates of muscle fibre numbers made from measurements of muscle cross-sectional area from CT images and muscle fibre area from biopsies, show that differences in size between trained and untrained men and women can all be accounted for by differences in muscle fibre size rather than fibre number.

In the pre-pubertal years, muscle strength in the quadriceps is related to the cube of height so that muscle strength increases in proportion to body mass and, consequently, the load the muscles have to support. Interestingly the biceps (a non-weight-bearing muscle group) increase in proportion to the square of the linear dimensions.[8] Since the strength of the major propulsive muscles increase in proportion to the load they have to propel, the ratio of strength to weight remains relatively constant throughout childhood and, on dimensional arguments, it might be predicted that there would be no change in performance.[10] Nevertheless, common experience of children, and measurements of performance, show a steady increase in running speed with a divergence between boys and girls at the age of puberty (**11.8**). Similar results have been obtained for other forms of activity[10] and illustrate, if nothing else, the considerable gap in our understanding of the biomechanical factors which determine physical performance in adults and children.

Power output

There is no doubt that success in the explosive athletic events, such as sprinting, jumping and throwing, requires a high muscular power output. The following sections will review the factors that determine power output. These conclusions are based largely on observations of adult muscle, although there is every reason to think that the same considerations apply to young muscle.

At the basic level of the muscle sarcomere, the force generated by the contractile elements depends on the number of actin and myosin filaments arranged in parallel, so that the isomeric force of human quadriceps is generally proportional to the cross sectional area of the muscle. But, within this relationship, there is a great deal of individual variation so that, overall, the cross-sectional area of a muscle explains only about half the difference in strength between people. Other factors determining the strength of a muscle include the level of activation and the speed and length of a muscle.

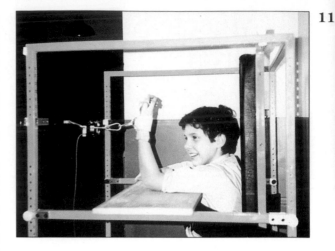

11.4 Measurement of muscle strength. A young boy about to test the strength of his forearm flexor muscles by pulling against the strain gauge attached to a cuff around his wrist. (See Parker *et al.*, 1990 for details).

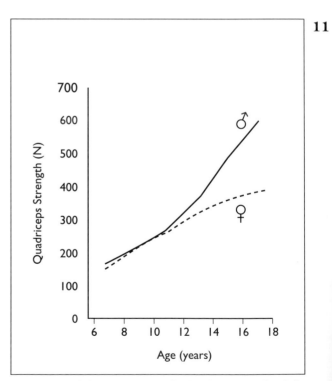

11.5 Quadriceps strength in boys and girls between 7 and 17 years. A cross-sectional survey of approximately 200 children of each sex carried out in two London schools (Parker *et al.*,1990).

.6

11.7

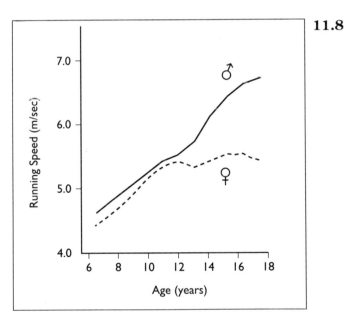

11.6, 11.7 Transverse sections of muscle biopsies taken from the quadriceps of a normal 35-year-old woman (**11.6**) and a normal 35-year-old man (**11.7**). Sections are stained with haematoxylin and eosin and photgraphed at the same magnification. Note the differences in size of the fibres between the sexes.

Activation

In the past, it has been widely thought that skeletal muscle cannot be fully activated by voluntary effort and there are many muscles over which the average person has little control, let alone can fully activate. The test of full activation is to compare the maximum voluntary contraction (MVC) force with that obtained by electrical stimulation of the muscle. This technique has been used to test the extent to which a variety of muscle groups can be activated by a voluntary effort. The general conclusion has been that, when tested individually, most major muscle groups used in athletic performance can be fully activated without training.[2] The technique of electrical stimulation has not been used systematically with children, and consequently there is no objective information as to whether they are able to fully activate their muscles. However, children over the age of about six show every sign of maximal effort, producing reproducible records, whilst younger children tend to be somewhat uncoordinated and unreliable in their efforts.[8]

Being able to fully activate a single muscle group is, however, only part of the story. It is known that healthy adults can fully activate their left and right biceps and that the strengths of the muscles are very similar, but most people can throw a ball much further with their dominant arm. The difference lies in the coordination of the many different muscle contractions which go to make up the entire movement.

11.8

11.8 Improvements in running speed with age. Cross-sectional data for North American children. from Hayden and Yahusz (1965), quoted by Shephard (1982).

The development of motor skills is outside the scope of this chapter but is an important factor determining the performance of a task, and a major factor determining athletic achievement of children. The effect of training in relation to skill and strength is discussed below.

Muscle length

As the angle of a joint alters, so the length of the muscle acting over that joint will also change. The arrangement of the contractile filaments in the sarcomere is such that changes in length give rise to changes in the force generated so that 'strength' has to be defined as the force generated in a particular position. Most activities require the muscles to work over a specific range of movement, and for maximum performance it would be advantageous for the muscles to be close to their optimum length at the time when they are making their contribution to the movement.

Skeletal muscle has the ability to change in overall length according to the position at which it is habitually used; lengthening or shortening occurs by the addition or loss of sarcomeres at the ends of the muscle fibres so that the average sarcomere length returns to a value close to the optimum for force generation. If a muscle is immobilised in a flexed position, a severe contracture can result and, by a similar mechanism, habitual training of muscles over a limited range of movement could well alter the overall length of the muscle and thus the force generated at a specific joint angle.

A number of studies have investigated the improvements in strength as a result of training at specific muscle lengths. The majority have found that the increases in strength are greatest with the limb in the position adopted during training[11], probably because of a change in the length of the muscle.

Speed of shortening

There is a characteristic relationship between speed of shortening and the force which a skeletal muscle can maintain (**11.9**), so that when considering the strength of a muscle it is necessary to specify the velocity of the movement as well as the length. The explosive movements of power athletes involve rapid muscular contraction so that the force developed during the movement will depend critically on the shape of the force/velocity curve. The main factor determining the shape of this relationship is the fibre type composition. Fast (type 2) fibres can produce considerably more force

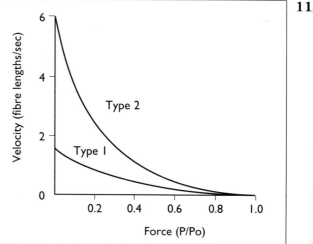

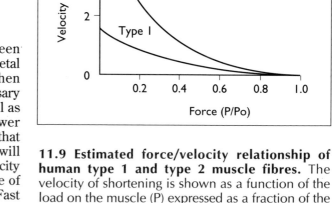

11.9 Estimated force/velocity relationship of human type 1 and type 2 muscle fibres. The velocity of shortening is shown as a function of the load on the muscle (P) expressed as a fraction of the maximum isometric force (P_0).

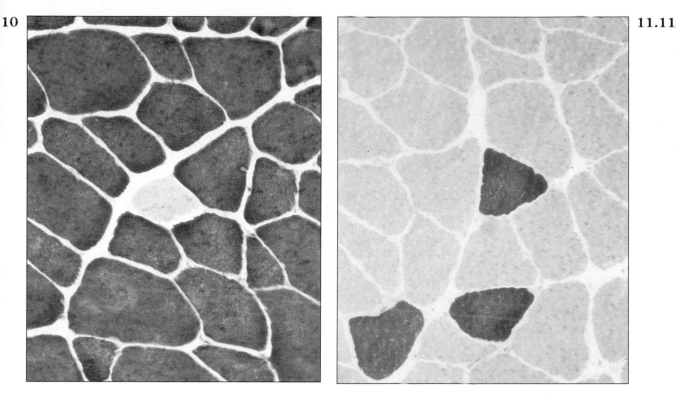

11.10, 11.11 Transverse sections of muscle biopsies taken from the quadriceps of a good high jumper (**11.10**) and a quality marathon runner (**11.11**). Sections were stained for myosin ATPase after preincubation at pH 9.4 so that the fast type 2 fibres stain dark and the slow type 1 fibres are pale. Note the difference in fibre composition between the two athletes.

than the slow (type 1) fibres when shortening at high velocities, even if they generate the same isometric force, and successful power athletes generally have a high proportion of type 2 fibres in their propulsive muscles (**11.10, 11.11**). Prolonged, relatively low force activity causes a change to slow contractile characteristics but the converse is not true. Prolonged, high frequency stimulation of cat muscle generating high forces caused a slowing of contractile characteristics similar to that seen with low frequency stimulation. It seems likely that any form of prolonged training, with high or low forces, will tend to make the muscles slower rather than increase power output.

The possibility of training for speed has received much attention, particularly since the advent of commercial isokinetic testing machines with reports of increases in strength which were greatest at, or near, the training velocities.[3,6] However, considerable caution must be observed in interpreting data obtained with isokinetic testing machines since the force/velocity relationships obtained are generally very flat and linear, bearing little resemblance to those obtained with isolated muscles or with human muscles *in situ.*

Connective tissue

Mammalian muscle fibres are enveloped in a connective tissue matrix which could have a role in transmitting tension to the tendons. Work-induced hypertrophy is known to increase collagen synthesis in animal muscle. An increase in the connective tissue content of a muscle, especially in the tendons, may be of value in storing potential energy during running and jumping, thereby making the movement more efficient, and this is one of the objectives of plyometric training. Such changes might not be termed, strictly, an increase in strength but, during exercise, the muscle and tendon should be considered as a functional unit.

Changes with training

Although most people undertaking a programme of weight training expect to develop larger and stronger muscles, most studies show that the achievements are limited to the performance of the specific training task and that there are relatively minor changes in the size and strength of individual muscles. Moreover, there is little or no benefit for other forms of exercise.[5]

One of the early indications that training was specific to the movement pattern was a study in which subjects trained the elbow flexors in the standing position and were subsequently assessed both standing and supine. The increase in muscle strength was much greater in the familiar than in an unfamiliar position. In a more recent study, subjects trained for 12 weeks by lifting near maximal loads on a leg extension machine.[5] After three months of training, the improvement in training load was of the order of 200% accompanied by only a 15% increase in the isometric strength of the quadriceps (**11.12**). Power output, assessed on a cycle ergometer, did not change over the twelve weeks.

Despite the improvement in the training exercise, there was no change in power output measured in the different task, even though the quadriceps was the main muscle group involved in both training and cycling. Such specificity suggests that the large increase in training weights lifted could be attributed to acquisition of skill in the training task, lifting weights, which was of little value when riding a bicycle. It is important to emphasise that performance is a combination of strength and skill and that skill is the factor most easily changed by training.

The relatively small change in strength of individual muscles is achieved with an even smaller increase in muscle size.[4] In the study described above, the increase in size was about 5% and barely significant (**11.13**). The reasons for the disproportionate increase in strength are not known but probably entail adaptations of muscle length, fibre pennation or connective tissue content. Studies of pre-pubertal children have come to very similar conclusions. A recent study[9] has shown improvements in strength and performance over the course of a 20-week training study with 9–11-year-old boys. There were no changes in the cross-sectional area of the muscles and the improvements were attributed to small changes in strength of individual muscles together with a more significant improvement in the coordination of the different muscle groups involved in the lifting tasks.

Motor skills are learned with relative ease in childhood and persist into adult life, whereas the

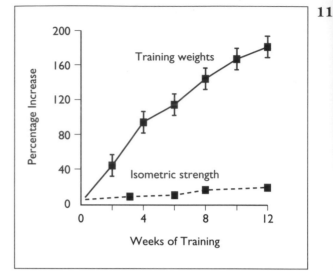

11.12 Improvements in weight training. A group of inexperienced subjects began training their quadriceps muscles and records were kept over 12 weeks of both the maximum training weights and the isometric strength of the quadriceps (Rutherford *et al.*, 1986). Note the discrepancy between the improvement in the training exercise and in the strength of the quadriceps.

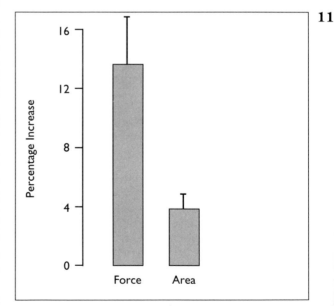

11.13 Improvements in weight training. In a similar study to that shown in **11.12**, the increase in strength and increase in muscle cross-sectional area were measured (Jones and Rutherford, 1987). Note that over 12 weeks training, the increase in strength was not matched by an increase in size of muscle.

adult has great difficulty in mastering new tasks. The acquisition of motor skills is probably the most valuable aspect of training for young athletes and it is important that the training they undertake is relevant to their own particular sport. Consequently, for the aspiring sprinter, time spent in weight training may well be of very limited value.

Despite the fact that most training studies seem to have shown increases in strength with little or no increase in muscle size, common experience tells us that prolonged heavy training or physical labour does lead to hypertrophy and increased strength of individual muscles in adults; the difference between experimental studies and real life is a question of time. Most experimental studies last only two or three months, but it appears that muscle hypertrophy occurs relatively slowly and requires several years of exercise before an obvious increase in size occurs. For the dedicated athlete, who has perfected his or her skills, increasing the muscle size represents the most obvious way forward. It is not clear whether habitual heavy exercise causes muscle hypertrophy in children. Not only are there no formal long-term training studies but any anecdotal information is complicated by the effects of normal growth. There are suggestions that prolonged activity may not have much effect. Maffulli[7] measured strength in elite young athletes and found that prepubertal boys were very similar in strength to sedentary boys while after puberty the athletes were significantly stronger. Athletic girls, however, were stronger than their sedentary counterparts at all ages.

The stimulus for muscle hypertrophy

A great deal has been written about the merits of different training protocols[1,5], but in many studies it is difficult to disentangle learning effects and possible neural adaptation from increases in strength and hypertrophy of individual muscles. Nevertheless, there is a general consensus that high forces have to be employed before any new muscle growth is obtained. At high forces both high (fast) and low (slow) threshold units are recruited and subjected to a training stimulus.

Exercise may result in endocrine or paracrine responses which stimulate muscle growth, but it is unlikely that endocrine changes are the major stimulus since hypertrophy is often limited to a single muscle group on one side of the body. Hormones, and especially testosterone, could have a permissive role in that a stimulus may be more effective in producing muscle hypertrophy if it is given in the presence of testosterone. For this reason, it is particularly important to carry out studies to determine whether muscle hypertrophy occurs to the same extent in men and women and in pre- and post-pubescent boys, but there is the problem of continuing a study for long enough to produce genuine muscle hypertrophy rather than simply improving skill and coordination.

Heavy exercise entails large metabolic fluxes with the accumulation of high concentrations of H^+, inorganic phosphate, creatine and other metabolites, and it is possible that one or more could stimulate muscle growth. However, these metabolite changes are associated with fatiguing rather than strengthening exercises and it is more likely that they would be the stimulus for mitochondrial proliferation and capillary growth, associated with increased endurance, rather than increase in muscle size and strength.

The other feature of heavy exercise is the high force developed in the muscle and tendons. High forces may lead to disruption of the Z disks causing myofibrils to split and the fragments to grow back to full size. Heavy exercise, especially that involving stretching active muscle, can cause more substantial damage to muscle fibres resulting in their degeneration and subsequent regeneration from activated satellite cells.

Training exercises in which muscles are stretched (eccentric exercise or negative work) can generate forces in the active muscles which are considerably greater than the more conventional exercise in which muscles shorten as weights are lifted. In addition, the metabolic costs are far less than during concentric work. A comparison of training using eccentric or concentric contractions should therefore provide a means of testing whether the stimulus for muscle growth is high force or metabolite changes. There has been one report that eccentric exercise is the best training stimulus but, perversely, the majority of studies which have used this approach have not shown a difference between the two types of exercise[4], and consequently the relative importance of force and metabolic change as stimuli for muscle growth remains unresolved.

Summary

The performance of any sporting activity involves a combination of skill and strength and it is very difficult to disentangle their separate contributions. The strength of an individual muscle depends on a number of factors. The major factor is the cross-sectional area of the muscle but others include the extent to which the muscle can be activated by voluntary effort, the overall length of the muscle and the position in which it is used, the fibre type composition and the velocity at which the movement takes place. Over a period of two or three months the major benefit of training is to improve the skill with which the training exercise is carried out. The effect is very specific so that there is considerable doubt as to whether weight training does anything other than train the athlete to lift weights. There is little doubt that, in this respect, children can train in the same way as adults and, as with adults, it is probably preferable that the children train using the motor skills involved in their own event rather than simply lifting weights. Increases in muscle size and strength in a healthy adult occur relatively slowly and, apart from the fact that high forces are required, little is known about the factors which stimulate growth. It would be surprising if children's muscles did not respond to increased use by increasing in size and strength but this has not been clearly demonstrated.

Acknowledgements

Our own work on growth of children has been supported by Action Research and the work on training by the Sports Council. We are grateful to Dr J.M. Round for providing the photographs.

References

1. Atha, J. (1981) Strengthening muscle. *Exerc. Sports Sci. Rev.* **9**: 1–73.
2. Bigland-Ritchie, B. and Woods, J.J. (1984) Changes in muscle contractile properties and neural control during human muscular fatigue. *Muscle Nerve* **7**: 691–699.
3. Caiozzo, V.J., Perrine, J.R., and Edgerton, V.R. (1981) Training induced alterations of the *in vivo* force-velocity relationship of human muscle. *J. Appl. Physiol.* **51**: 750–754.
4. Jones, D.A. and Rutherford, O.M. (1987) Human muscle strength training: the effects of three different training regimes and the nature of the resultant changes. *J. Physiol.* **391**: 1–11.
5. Jones, D.A., Rutherford, O.M. and Parker, D.F. (1989) Physiological changes in skeletal muscle as a result of strength training. *Quart. J. Exp. Physiol.* **74**: 233–256.
6. Kanehisa, H. and Miyashita, M. (1983) Specificity of velocity in strength training. *Eur. J. Appl. Physiol.* **52**: 104–106.
7. Maffulli, N. (1992) *The effects of intensive training on the musculo-skeletal system of elite young athletes.* PhD Thesis, University of London.
8. Parker, D.F., Round, J.M., Sacco, P. and Jones, D.A. (1990) A cross-sectional survey of upper and lower limb strength in boys and girls during childhood and adolescence. *Ann. Human Biol.* **17**: 199–211.
9. Ramsay, J.A., Blimkie, C.J.R., Smith, K., Garner, S., MacDougall, J.D. and Sale, D. (1990) Strength training effects in prepubescent boys. *Med. Sci. Sports Exerc.* **22**: 605–614.
10. Shephard, R.J. (1982) *Physical activity and growth.* Year Book Medical Publishers Inc., Chicago.
11. Thepaut-Mathieu, C., Hoecke, J. and Maton, B. (1988) Myoelectrical and mechanical changes linked to length specificity during isometric training. *J. Appl. Physiol.* **64**: 1500–1505.

12. Laboratory Testing of Young Athletes

Neil Armstrong and Joanne Welsman

Purposes

A well-constructed laboratory testing programme can be used to indicate a young athlete's strengths and weaknesses and to enable suitable training regimes to be designed. Progress may be monitored and alterations to training programmes made on the basis of laboratory test results. Problem areas associated with potential injury may be identified. The results of appropriate laboratory tests may be used to monitor rehabilitation procedures and to make decisions on whether a young athlete is ready to return to his or her sport. The laboratory may provide an educational environment in which sports scientist, young athlete and coach can interact to increase understanding of how the body responds to exercise and adapts to training.

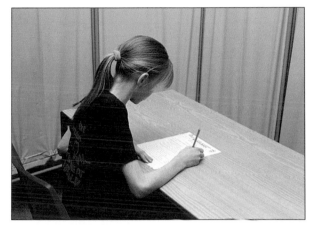

12.1 Pre-test health screen questionnaire. Should be completed prior to exercise.

Limitations

Laboratory tests should not be used to identify future Olympians during their youth as genetic limits to the potential to improve are largely unknown. Team selection should not be based solely on physiological tests as performance is often an interaction of tactical, technical, psychological and physiological elements. It is often difficult to simulate sports performance in a laboratory and the value of non-sport-specific tests decreases as the motor patterns tested become more removed from the actual performance. Testing equipment may also be a problem with young athletes and the influence of using respiratory valves, tubing and mixing chambers designed for use with adults needs further evaluation.

Ethics

With minors, it is particularly important to obtain informed consent from both the athlete and his/her parents. It is necessary and desirable that young athletes involved in a laboratory testing programme

fully understand the implications, to themselves, of the procedures to which they are consenting. It should be stressed that they are free to terminate any of the procedures when they wish. Many of the invasive procedures used with consenting adults (e.g. muscle biopsies) are not appropriate for use with minors.

Pre-test preparation

It is essential that all tests are carried out under standardised conditions in a stable laboratory environment. Young athletes should maintain their normal diet prior to the day of testing and eat only a light carbohydrate meal at least two hours before any test procedure. Only light training should be carried out on the day before testing, and on test-day young athletes should not exercise prior to their laboratory visit.

On their first visit to the laboratory young athletes may be anxious. They should therefore be given adequate explanation of the proposed protocols and objectives and gradually habituated to the exercise procedures. A health screen questionnaire should be completed and interpreted

12.2

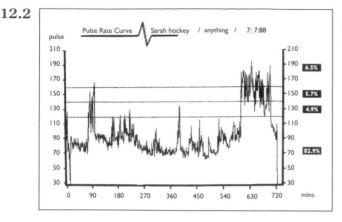

12.2 Habitual physical activity estimated from 12 hour continuous heart rate monitoring. Training sessions may be easily identified.

12

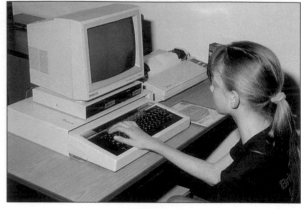

12.3 Computer analysis of diet diary.

12

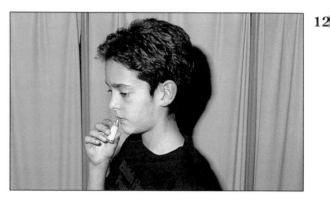

12.4 Collection of a saliva sample for subsequent testosterone analysis.

before testing takes place. Athletes suffering from viral infections should not be allowed to participate in laboratory tests. Nutritional and habitual physical activity data may be obtained through pre-test questionnaires or, preferably, from diet diaries and continuous heart rate monitoring carried out before the laboratory visit.

Kinanthropometry

In kinanthropometry, measurements are used to appraise size, shape, proportion, composition and maturation. Kinanthropometric measurements are vital if young athletes' performances are to be objectively analysed. Chronological age should be recorded in decimal fractions of years. The rating of secondary sex characteristics provides a useful index of maturity. Tanner's five point rating of pubic hair, breast and genital development is the most common procedure. In girls, the age of menarche should be noted and, in boys, salivary testosterone level may provide useful information.

Height and weight should be recorded but the use of height to weight indices (e.g. body mass index) as measures of body composition is not recommended. Young athletes often have a relatively high body mass index through the possession of a large musculoskeletal system rather than extra fat. Girths (e.g. chest, waist, thigh) and breadths (e.g. biacromial, biiliocristal) are valuable ancillary measures.

12.5

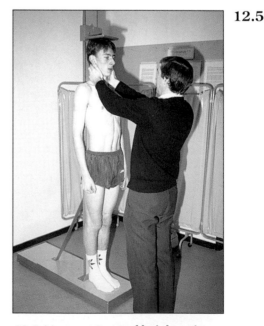

12.5 Measurement of height using a stadiometer.

Skinfold thicknesses are useful indicators of children's body fatness but should be used as raw scores as the accurate interpretation of young athletes' skinfold data in terms of body fatness cannot be made at the present time. Skinfolds should be taken on the same side of the body, normally the right, and common skinfold thicknesses include triceps, biceps, supra-iliac, subscapular, abdominal, front thigh and medial calf.

Densitometry is widely acknowledged as the criterion method of measuring body density. Its use with young athletes is complicated by the fact that growth and development evoke changes in body composition that affect the conceptual basis for estimating fatness and leanness. Some solutions and tabulations of fat-free body composition density in children and youth as reference values are available.[1] Bioelectrical impedance is a recently developed method of estimating body composition.

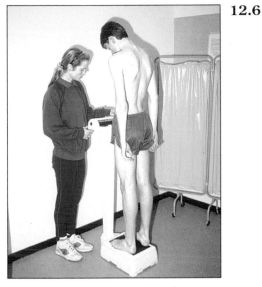

12.6

12.6 Measurement of body mass using balance beam scales.

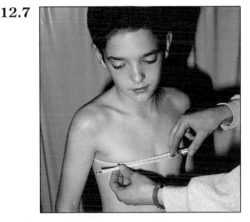

12.7

12.7 Chest circumference. One of several girths which may be measured. Others include relaxed arm, flexed arm, forearm, wrist, ankle, calf, thigh, waist and gluteal.

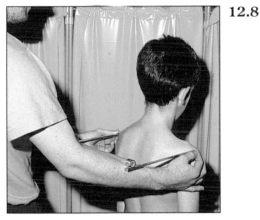

12.8

12.8 Biacromial breadth. One of several breadths of interest. Others include chest, biiliocristal, epicondylar humerus width and epicondylar femur width.

12.9 **12.10** **12.11**

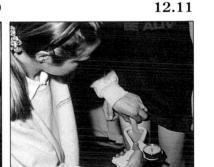

12.9–12.11 Triceps, biceps, thigh skinfolds measurement. Other common skinfold thicknesses include supra-iliac, subscapular and medial calf.

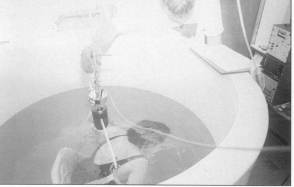

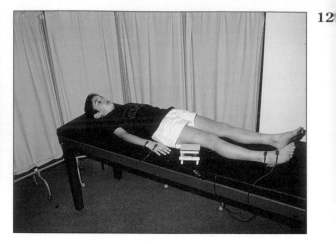

12.12 Densitometry is widely acknowledged as the criterion measure of body composition but its use with children is problematic.

12.13 Bioelectrical impedance is a simple, rapid method of estimating body composition which is growing in popularity.

Initial results have been promising and its use in sports science laboratories is likely to increase. The introduction of magnetic resonance imaging into some laboratories has enabled non-invasive analyses of young athletes' fat distribution.[2]

Bioenergetics

Exercise requires energy and the energy to support muscular contraction is produced during the splitting of the high energy phosphates, primarily adenosine triphosphate (ATP). The quantity of ATP stored in the muscles is very small, perhaps sufficient to sustain maximal exercise for about 1s. ATP must therefore be re-generated if activity is to continue beyond this time. Initially, it is provided through the splitting of another high energy phosphate, creatine phosphate. Unfortunately, maximal exercise can only be exclusively supported in this manner for a further 4–5s as muscular stores of creatine phosphate are also limited. Muscular concentration of high energy phosphates is similar in adults, adolescents and children although if the child's smaller muscle mass is considered it can be seen that the young subject has a smaller total reservoir of high energy phosphates than the adult. Muscle biopsy studies have indicated that the relative depletion of high energy phosphate stores during exhausting exercise proceeds at much the same relative rate between 12 and 23 years of age.

Glycogenolysis is initiated well before high energy phosphate stores are maximally depleted and ATP is re-synthesised during the catabolism of glycogen to pyruvic acid and subsequently to lactic

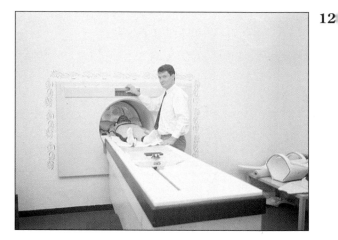

12.14 Fat distribution may be analysed through magnetic resonance imaging.

acid. Children and adolescents do not seem to be as well equipped as adults in generating energy via the glycogenolytic system. Although it has been suggested that this is due to reduced activities of glycolytic enzymes such as phosphofructokinase, this diminished anaerobic capacity probably reflects children's overall muscle metabolic profile in which the ratio of oxidative to glycolytic enzymes is greater than in adults.

ATP re-synthesis through either the splitting of creatine phosphate or the catabolism of glycogen to lactic acid does not require the presence of oxygen. These systems are therefore called anaerobic energy systems. During prolonged activity, however, the individual's performance depends largely upon his/her ability to deliver oxygen to the working muscles. This aerobic system is the most efficient in terms of ATP production, and has a much greater capacity for energy generation than the anaerobic systems. The oxygen transport system is slow to adapt to the demands of heavy exercise, and the rate at which ATP can be generated through glycolysis/glycogenolysis in muscle greatly exceeds that of the aerobic system. As a result, near the beginning of the exercise, when the mitochondrial oxygen consumption is not optimal, and during very intense exercise, when pyruvic acid production exceeds the mitochondrial capacity to oxidise it, anaerobic glycogenolysis is of primary importance.

If a total picture of responses to exercise is required, both the anaerobic and aerobic processes must be considered. The relative importance of the energy systems and their analysis is dependent upon the young athlete's sporting role or event. Young athletes capable of high anaerobic performance may not have a similar aerobic potential and laboratory assessment will provide valuable insights.

Aerobic performance

Maximal oxygen uptake

Maximal oxygen uptake ($\dot{V}O_2$max) is defined as the maximum rate at which an individual can consume oxygen whilst breathing air at sea level. It provides an overview of the function of the oxygen transport system and reflects pulmonary, cardiovascular and muscular components. The measurement of $\dot{V}O_2$max requires the subject to exercise to exhaustion. Several investigators have been reluctant to carry out this type of test with children and adolescents, and have therefore attempted to predict it from submaximal data. There is, however, no valid substitute for a direct determination of $\dot{V}O_2$max.[3]

The principal criterion of $\dot{V}O_2$max, having been reached during a laboratory test, is that there is no further increase in oxygen uptake despite an increase in exercise intensity i.e. the demonstration of a $\dot{V}O_2$max plateau. However, only a minority of children and adolescents exhibit a true $\dot{V}O_2$max plateau. It appears that there is often no tendency for oxygen consumption to level off despite maximal efforts by young male or female athletes. In our laboratory, all maximal tests with children and adolescents are terminated by voluntary exhaustion, i.e. when the child, despite strong

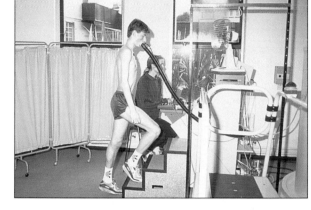

12.15

12.15 Step tests are often terminated by local muscle fatigue rather than cardiopulmonary factors.

verbal encouragement from the experimenters, is unwilling or unable to continue. We therefore prefer to use the term 'peak $\dot{V}O_2$', which represents the highest oxygen uptake elicited during an exercise test to exhaustion. If the subject has been habituated to the testing procedures and environment, his/her peak heart rate either levels off several minutes prior to the final exercise intensity or reaches a value at least 95% of age predicted maximal heart rate, and his/her respiratory exchange ratio exceeds unity, we accept peak $\dot{V}O_2$ as a maximal index.

The choice of laboratory ergometer for the measurement of peak $\dot{V}O_2$ generally lies between step bench, cycle ergometer and treadmill. It is difficult to persuade young athletes to climb a step with a consistent rhythm and problems may arise from differences in leg length. The major drawback is the young subject's lack of mass. In our experience, stepping exercise with children and adolescents is seldom terminated by cardiopulmonary insufficiency and peak $\dot{V}O_2$ is about 25% lower than that elicited during cycle ergometry. The treadmill engages a larger muscle mass in the exercise than the cycle ergometer, and the peak $\dot{V}O_2$ obtained is therefore more likely to be limited by central rather than peripheral factors. In cycle ergometry, a high proportion of the total power output is developed by the quadriceps muscle and the effort required is large in relation to muscle strength. Blood flow through the quadriceps is limited, resulting in increased anaerobic metabolism and consequent termination of exercise by peripheral muscle pain. Treadmill-determined peak

12.16

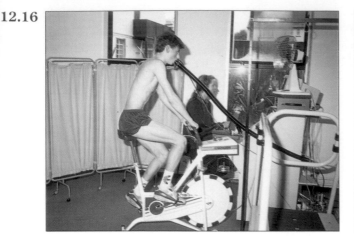

12.16 Peak oxygen uptake may be determined using cycle ergometry but values are about 10% lower than those elicited on a treadmill.

12.1[

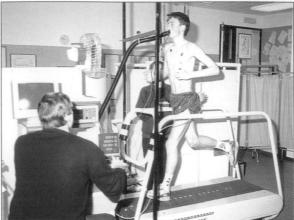

12.17 The treadmill is the ergometer of choice as peak oxygen uptake is more likely to be limited by central rather than peripheral factors.

12.18

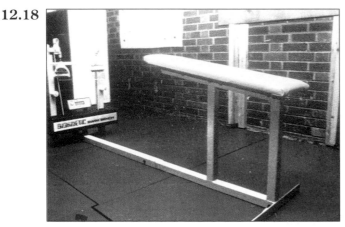

12.18 It is important to simulate athletes' competitive performance in the laboratory. Biokinetic swimbenches may be useful for testing young swimmers.

$\dot{V}O_2$ values are about 9% higher than cycle ergometer values. The treadmill is therefore generally the machine of choice although some ancillary measures are easier to obtain during cycle ergometry. It is, however, important to simulate athletes' competitive performance as closely as possible, and a treadmill may not always be appropriate. Very little valid feedback can be given to a coach if his/her swimmers are tested on a treadmill.

It seems that, regardless of the ergometer utilised, the experimental protocol is not critical and

peak $\dot{V}O_2$ is very reproducible if subjects are well-motivated. The advantage of a continuous protocol is that it is less time consuming but a discontinuous test enables easier measurement of ancillary parameters such as blood lactate. In general, we favour a discontinuous, incremental protocol with three minute exercise bouts interspersed with one minute rest periods, but the optimum protocol for a young athlete simulates the demands of his/her competitive performance.

Absolute peak $\dot{V}O_2$ (measured in $l.min^{-1}$) increases steadily throughout childhood and adolescence. Therefore, in order to compare the peak $\dot{V}O_2$ of two athletes of different body mass or to monitor changes in peak $\dot{V}O_2$ within the same athlete over a period of training, it is conventional to express the measure in mass-related terms, i.e. $ml.kg^{-1}.min^{-1}$. It is well documented that mass-related peak $\dot{V}O_2$ shows little change during childhood and adolescence in boys, although in untrained girls there tends to be a decline.[3]

There has been much debate as to whether the expression of peak $\dot{V}O_2$ as a ratio with body mass adequately partitions out differences in body size. The major criticism of this approach is that it fails to account for the linear relationship which exists between peak $\dot{V}O_2$ and body mass in addition to that between peak $\dot{V}O_2$ and age. The generation of regression lines based upon the relationship between body mass and absolute peak $\dot{V}O_2$ ($l.min^{-1}$) at different ages or stages of maturation during growth may represent a more appropriate method by which an individual's peak $\dot{V}O_2$ can be compared against the norms for a specific population.[4] For

12.19 The generation of regression standards allows comparison of peak $\dot{V}O_2$ independently of body dimensions such as height and mass. This figure illustrates the difference in peak $\dot{V}O_2$ between 10- and 15-year-old boys which conventional analysis fails to identify.

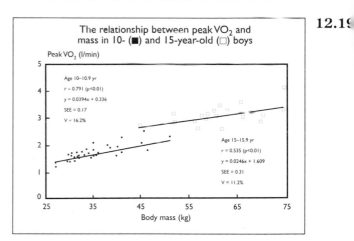

example, using this type of analysis it can be shown that peak $\dot{V}O_2$ of 10-year-old boys is lower than that of 15-year-old boys, perhaps reflecting increased haemoglobin levels and muscle mass in the older boys.[5] This contrasts with the conventional comparison of ratio standards which fail to demonstrate a difference over this age range.

An alternative approach has applied dimensionality theory to the interpretation of growth-related changes in peak $\dot{V}O_2$. This assumes that body segments remain in the same proportion to one another during growth. Changes in body dimensions and physiological variables can thus be predicted from changes in body length (L). Using this theory, peak $\dot{V}O_2$ should be scaled to L^2. Others have suggested that an exponent of 2 is incorrect and values ranging from 1.51 to 3.21 have been applied. Therefore, this approach also has considerable limitations.

The concept of metabolic scope offers another means of examining aerobic capacity changes in the child or adolescent athlete independently of body dimensions. Metabolic scope describes the magnitude of increase from resting to peak $\dot{V}O_2$. In adult athletes, maximal oxygen uptake may represent a 15-fold increase above basal values. In contrast, children are able to elicit only a 10-fold increase.[6]

Serial measures of lung function, pulmonary diffusing capacity, haemoglobin concentration and haematocrit are informative and are measured routinely in many sports science laboratories. Heart rate is relatively easy to monitor accurately and an estimate of cardiac output enables stroke volume (cardiac output = heart rate × stroke volume) and arterial-venous oxygen difference (oxygen uptake = cardiac output × arterial-venous oxygen difference) to be calculated. Young athletes' cardiac output may be estimated from acetylene rebreathing, electrical bioimpedance or the Doppler frequency shift, but the indirect Fick method involving carbon dioxide

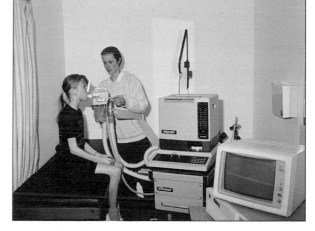

12.20 Diffusion capacity may be determined using the carbon monoxide single breath method. It is a valuable measure for swimmers.

rebreathing is probably the best suited for exercise cardiac output determination.[7] The indirect carbon dioxide technique has been incorporated into automated exercise testing systems and the values of cardiac output compare favourably with both dye dilution and direct Fick measurements.

The use of Borg's Rating of Perceived Exertion (RPE) may provide valuable supplementary information over a series of laboratory visits.[8]

In addition to measuring peak $\dot{V}O_2$, many laboratories now routinely supplement this maximal measure with submaximal markers of cardio-pulmonary fitness and aerobic endurance capacity. Changes in the blood lactate response to an incremental exercise test provide perhaps the most sensitive measure of an athlete's capacity for aerobic endurance performance. These changes are particularly valuable for detecting performance

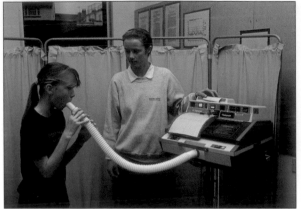

12.21 Dynamic lung volumes such as forced vital capacity and forced expiratory volume may be easily determined using a vitalograph.

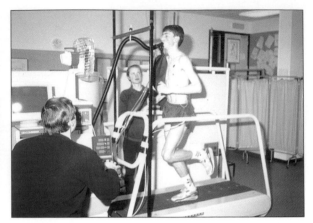

12.22 Carbon dioxide re-breathing is probably the best method for exercise cardiac output determination.

improvements in the highly-trained individual who is unable to elicit further increases in peak $\dot{V}O_2$.

During the initial stages of an incremental exercise, test blood lactate levels show little increase as processes of lactate production and removal, although increased, remain balanced. As intensity increases further, this equilibrium is lost, lactate production outstrips removal, and blood lactate levels increase exponentially to produce the typical curve. Improvements in muscle oxidative capacity with training allow athletes to exercise at higher relative exercise intensities before a progressive accumulation of lactate in muscle and blood occurs, thus shifting the blood lactate response curve to the right.

The point at which the rapid increase in blood lactate levels occurs has been termed the 'anaerobic threshold'. This point was suggested to represent a limitation in oxygen supply to the muscle cell and consequent onset of anaerobic metabolism, although this assumption has been extensively challenged. Because of the close correspondence between the blood lactate curve and the ventilatory response during a progressive exercise test with stages of 30s–1 min, it has been common to attempt to identify this point from changes in ventilation or gas exchange variables. However, this method is not recommended, as the two curves may be dissociated under a number of conditions, for example, glycogen depletion. In children, where breathing patterns may be erratic, the ventilatory inflection point may be particularly difficult to detect.[3]

Direct measures of blood lactate during exercise testing are, therefore, preferable. Incremental

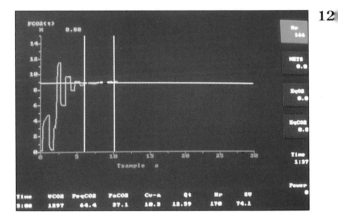

12.23 The carbon dioxide rebreathing technique has been incorporated into several automated exercise testing systems.

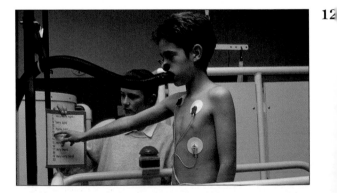

12.24 Borg's Rating of Perceived Exertion (RPE) may provide valuable information over a series of laboratory visits.

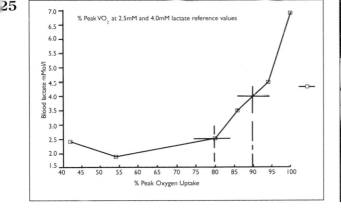

12.25 | 12.26

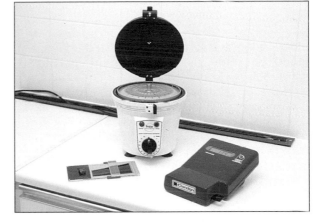

12.25 Interpolation of the exercise intensity at fixed blood lactate reference values provides an objective assessment of aerobic endurance capacity.

12.26 Blood collection from the fingertip is recommended for the determination of lactate, glucose and cholesterol during a laboratory test.

12.27

12.27 Haemoglobin and Haematocrit should be routinely monitored in young athletes, particularly females.

stages of at least three minutes are recommended for young athletes in order for blood lactate levels to accurately reflect the exercise intensity being performed. In preference to the subjective detection of the exercise intensity at the point of inflection in the lactate curve, performance corresponding to a fixed blood lactate reference value may be interpolated. With adult athletes, a fixed blood lactate reference value of 4.0 mmol.l^{-1} is recommended. However, as children demonstrate much lower blood lactates during exercise, this level often ceases to be submaximal, and a reference value of 2.5 mmol.l^{-1} is more appropriate.[9] The recommendation for this lower value is supported by the finding that the maximal level of blood lactate which can be sustained without a progressive increase during prolonged exercise (i.e. the maximal lactate steady state) tends to occur at approximately 2.5 mmol.l^{-1} in adolescents.[10]

The site of sampling and the assay medium are two methodological aspects of blood lactate measurement which may significantly alter the blood lactate/exercise intensity relationship, and so require consideration during the interpretation and or comparison of an athlete's test results.[11]

Blood samples for lactate assay may be drawn from arteries (radial or brachial), veins (antecubital or dorsal hand vein), or capillaries (fingertip or earlobe). During incremental cycle ergometry, lactate levels in venous blood tend to be lower than in arterial blood, with the difference increasing at higher intensities. However, during treadmill exercise with stages of 3–4 min, arterial/venous blood lactate differences are less pronounced.

Arterial or venous sampling are not recommended for routine use with young athletes in non-clinical

settings as catheterisation is required. However, arterial lactate levels are well reflected in capillary blood from either the fingertip or earlobe, providing that blood flow to the sampling site is maintained, usually by the application of heat. As capillary sampling requires less technical expertise than sampling from other sites, and is less traumatic to the subject, its use is recommended with young athletes.

Most of the modern semi-automatic, portable lactate analysers assay lactate in the plasma fraction of whole blood, i.e. the blood sample entered into the analyser contains both the solid (mainly the red

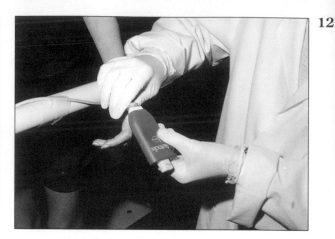

12.28 An automatic analyser provides glucose and lactate measurements from a single 25 μl blood sample within 60 seconds.

12.29 Automatic lancing devices which prevent the accidental re-use of a needle are recommended for fingertip blood sampling.

blood cells) and liquid (plasma) components of blood but only the lactate in the plasma is measured.

However, other analysers require different blood preparations such as plasma, or lysed blood (blood which has been chemically treated to break down red cells, thus releasing intracellular lactate). Lactate levels measured in lysed blood are slightly higher than those in whole blood, with the difference increasing at higher concentrations of lactate. This difference reflects the addition of the cellular lactate to the assay in the lysed blood sample. Plasma lactate levels are higher than both lysed and whole blood by approximately 30%. If the same volume of either whole blood or plasma is passed into the analyser, then the actual volume of plasma assayed in the whole blood sample is smaller than in the plasma-only sample due to the presence of cellular components of the blood. As a result, the lactate level measured is lower.

These differences become important if the blood lactate/exercise intensity relationship is to be used to indicate appropriate training intensities. The pattern of increase in lactate observed in plasma will be shifted to the left of the curve based upon whole blood and, therefore, a given level of lactate will represent a considerably lower exercise intensity compared with that based upon whole blood.

Because of these differences, athletes should be tested under standardised conditions using the same sampling and assay techniques. Caution should be applied when comparing the results with other athletes whose conditions of testing may have been different.

Blood sampling during the physiological assessment of an athlete inevitably carries some risk of cross-infection between technician and athlete. Therefore, the safety aspects of blood sampling are of primary importance and a strict safety code should be adhered to. Protective clothing and gloves should be worn by the technician during blood sampling and handling procedures. The athlete's finger should be lanced with a device which does not permit the accidental re-use of a needle. All contaminated material including needles, capillary tubes/cuvettes, swabs, gloves etc. should be disposed of in appropriately marked sharps bins and containers for incineration. Any accidental skin punctures should be reported to a medical practitioner.

Anaerobic performance

The ability to repeatedly produce a high power output for a short period of time is fundamental to many sports. However, despite their predominance during maximal efforts of short duration, the testing of the anaerobic energy systems is not as well advanced as aerobic testing and sport-specific laboratory tests are often difficult to design. The Margaria Step Test is probably the most well established test of short-term anaerobic performance. This involves measuring the speed at which the young athlete can run up a staircase of known

12.30

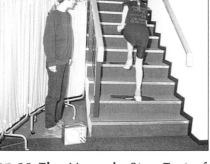

12.30 The Margaria Step Test of short-term anaerobic performance relies on high energy phosphates.

12.31

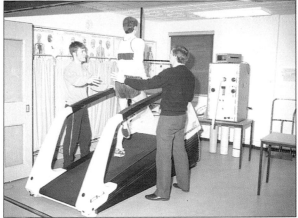

12.31 The Cunningham and Faulkner Treadmill Test relies heavily on subject motivation to do well.

12.32

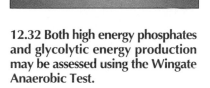

12.32 Both high energy phosphates and glycolytic energy production may be assessed using the Wingate Anaerobic Test.

height. Several variations of this test are available, and all rely heavily on high energy phosphate stores.

The glycolytic system may be taxed using the Cunningham and Faulkner Treadmill Test. This test consists of running on a treadmill up a 20% gradient at 3.56 m.s^{-1}. The time to exhaustion is noted and post-exercise blood lactate is often recorded. The test relies heavily on the subject's motivation to do well.

The most sensitive and reliable assessment of anaerobic performance is probably provided by variants of the Wingate Anaerobic Test.[8] Both high energy phosphates and glycolytic energy production can be assessed using the Wingate Test. In its original form, the test consisted of pedalling or arm cranking as fast as possible for 30s against a known constant resistance. Performance was expressed by three indices, peak power (defined as the highest power output in a 5s period), mean power (defined as the mean work output over the 30s period), and fatigue index (defined as the difference between the peak power and the lowest 5s power output divided by peak power). More recent applications of the Wingate Test have employed multiple short test protocols either to optimise peak power output or to simulate the repeated short sprints basic to many sports.[12] Isokinetic cycling tests and non-motorised treadmill runs have been devised to assess anaerobic performance, but the Wingate Anaerobic Test using a friction-braked cycle ergometer remains the most secure.

12.33

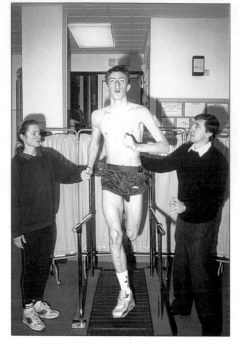

12.34

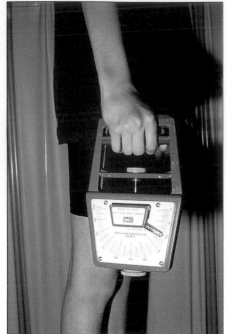

12.33 Anaerobic performance may be assessed from sprints on a non-motorised treadmill interfaced with a micro-computer.

12.34 Isometric dynamometry. Measurement of hand grip strength.

Strength and flexibility

Most laboratory testing of young athletes focuses on aerobic and anaerobic performance, but other important components of performance include strength and flexibility. Strength is commonly measured in sports science laboratories using isometric contractions. Hand grip, leg and back dynamometers are readily available. Weight lifting strength (i.e. the heaviest weight that can be lifted once through a specified range of movement) often supplements isometric measures. Well-equipped laboratories may use isokinetic dynamometers which provide resistance by accommodating the force or torque applied against the resistance mechanism, and thus preventing acceleration beyond the set velocity of movement. The best strength test is the one most specific to the young athlete's competitive sport.

Flexibility, the range of motion about a joint or a series of joints, may be measured using still photography, cinematography, videotape, goniometry and electrogoniometry but, due to financial and time constraints, the Leighton Flexometer is probably still the instrument of choice in most sports science laboratories. The flexometer consists

12.35

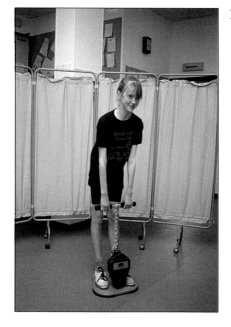

12.35 Isometric dynamometry. Measurement of back strength.

36

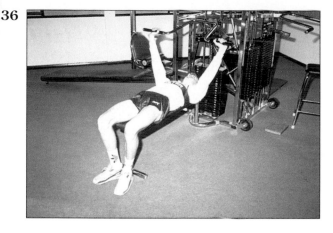

12.37

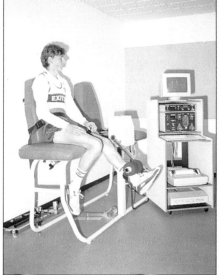

12.36 Weight lifting to determine the one repetition maximum.

12.37 Isokinetic dynamometry. The provision of resistance by accommodating the force of torque applied against the resistance mechanism and thus preventing acceleration beyond the set velocity of movement.

of a weighted 360° dial and a weighted pointer mounted in a case. The dial and pointer operate freely and independently, the movement of each being controlled by gravity. Independent locking devices stop all movement of either the pointer or dial at any given position. While in use, the flexometer is strapped to the segment being tested. It has been shown to be a reliable instrument for measuring static flexibility at several joints.[13]

12.38

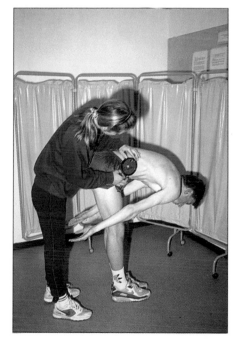

Summary

If appropriate, well-controlled laboratory tests are repeated at regular intervals and the results are reported promptly to the athlete and coach, and interpreted in language they can understand. A mutually beneficial partnership between athlete, coach and sports scientist should evolve. The laboratory results will enhance the information available to the coach and facilitate the optimum development of his young athletes.

Acknowledgement

We are grateful to Bryan D. Woods for assisting in the preparation of photographs.

12.38 Estimation of flexibility using the Leighton Flexometer.

References

1. Lohman, T.G. (1989) Assessment of body composition in children. *Pediatr. Exerc. Sc.* **1**: 19–30.
2. Peters, D., Fox, K., Armstrong, N., Sharpe, P., and Bell, M. (1994) Support from magnetic resonance imaging for skinfold estimates of adiposity in 11-year old children. *Amer. J. Hum. Biol.* **6**:237–243.
3. Armstrong, N., and Welsman, J. (1994) Assessment and interpretation of aerobic fitness in children and adolescents. *Exerc. Sports Sci. Revs.* **22**:435–476.
4. Tanner, J.M. (1989) Fallacy of per-weight and per-surface area standards and their relation to spurious correlation. *J. Appl. Physiol.* **2**: 1–15.
5. Williams, J., Armstrong, N., Winter, E. and Crichton, N. (1992) Changes in peak oxygen uptake with age and sexual maturation in boys: physiological fact or statistical anomaly? *Children and Exercise XVI.* 35–37.
6. Rowland, T.W. (1991) 'Normalising' maximal oxygen uptake, or the search for the Holy Grail (per kg). *Pediatr. Exerc. Sci.* **3**: 95–102.
7. Driscoll, D.J., Staats, B.A. and Beck, K.C. (1989) Measurement of cardiac output in children during exercise: a review. *Pediatr. Exerc. Sci.* **1**: 102–115.
8. Bar-Or, O. (1983) *Paediatric Sports Medicine for the Practitioner.* Springer-Verlag, New York.
9. Williams, J. and Armstrong, N. (1991) The influence of age and sexual maturation on children's blood lactate responses to exercise. *Pediatr. Exerc. Sci.* **3**: 111–120.
10. Williams, J. and Armstrong, N. (1991) The maximal lactate steady state and its relationship to performance at fixed blood lactate reference values in children. *Pediatr. Exerc. Sci.* **3**: 333–341.
11. Williams, J., Armstrong, N. and Kirby, B. (1992) The influence of site of sampling and assay medium upon the measurement and interpretation of blood lactate responses to exercise. *J. Sports Sci.* **10**:95–107.
12. Winter, E.M. (1991) Cycle ergometry and maximal exercise. *Sports Med.* **11**: 351–357.
13. MacDougall, J.D., Wenger, H.A. and Green, H.J. (Eds) (1991) *Physiological Testing of the High-Performance Athlete.* Human Kinetics, Champaign, Il.

13 Field Testing in Young Athletes

Francesco Conconi, Chiara Borsetto
and Elena Ballarin

Numerous field tests are currently being used for the functional evaluation of children and adolescents. In an attempt to standardize these tests, the European Council, Committee for Sports Development proposed in 1988 the Eurofit programme[5], which describes several protocols for carrying out functional evaluations in children and adolescents. The proposed tests take into consideration various aspects of physical capacity, including cardiorespiratory endurance, strength, muscular endurance, speed, flexibility, and balance. The aim of the Eurofit programme is 'to invite children to enjoy regular participation in sports and other physical activities' but 'not ... to provide an early talent-spotting system or to put emphasis on competition.' Therefore, the programme may be useful for collecting data on physiological characteristics and attitudes towards various sports among the student population, but it is too general and not designed for gathering information on youths already involved in competitive sports.

Trainers from individual sports have their athletes carry out specific field tests that provide information on performance capacities in that sport. These tests have both practical importance and physiological significance. Yet the variety of tests in use, and the lack of a systematic study of test results prevent the proposal of any single field test for evaluating young athletes.

We consider it appropriate to propose in this Atlas four field tests suitable for evaluating the basic physiological characteristics of young athletes. The described field tests are not specific to various sports but are based upon running, an action that is simple and feasible for whatever sport the athlete may practise. In this respect they are similar to commonly used laboratory tests that evaluate not specific physiological characteristics, but the athlete's basic characteristics through the performance of simple movements such as running on a treadmill or pedalling on a bicycle ergometer.

The tests described here, which have been systematically applied to adults, adolescents and children, allow for the evaluation of:

- Acceleration and maximal speed, an expression of neuromuscular power and the power output of the anaerobic mechanisms.

- Speed at the anaerobic threshold, that is, the maximal power output of the aerobic mechanism without the use of the anaerobic lactacid mechanism.
- Maximal speed obtained with the activation of the anaerobic lactacid mechanism, disaggregated from the other mechanisms of ATP resynthesis.
- We also describe the Cooper test, a field test often used, that, in contrast to the above three tests, does not allow a reductive analysis of a single mechanism but provides an overall evaluation of the two principal energy mechanisms, used simultaneously, i.e. aerobic and anaerobic lactacid metabolism.

Test for acceleration and maximal speed

This test evaluates maximal neuromuscular and metabolic power, primarily of the lower limb muscles. It requires particular concentration, and good results can be obtained only by having the subject repeat the test often enough so that it becomes habitual. The brevity of the test almost completely excludes the aerobic mechanism and also excludes an accumulation of lactate great enough to interfere with the efficiency of muscular contraction.

Test procedure

A good warm-up prior to the test is indispensable for optimal results and helps to prevent muscular damage that can be caused by maximal efforts from a cold start. The test is performed on a linear 30m section of an athletic track that is divided into three 10m sections (**13.1**). The test subject starts from an erect position with his right foot exactly behind the starting line. He is instructed to run the 30m at the maximal speed possible. Three times are registered by means of photocells placed every 10m, and the corresponding speeds are calculated. The test is repeated three times with 5min rest

13.1

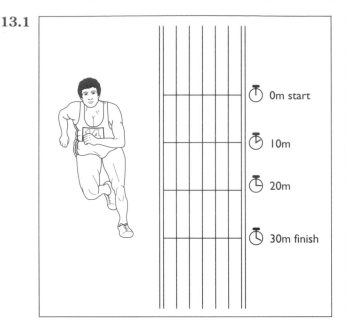

13.1 Test for acceleration and maximal speed. Procedure.

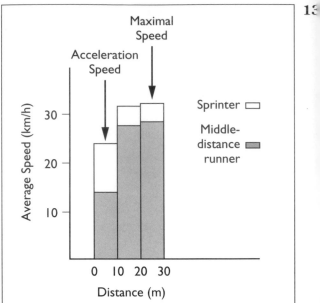

13.2 Test for acceleration and maximal speed. Results.

intervals between tests. If more detailed information is desired, the course may divided into smaller sections with the use of additional photocells.

Results

Figure **13.2** shows the results obtained by a sprinter and by a middle-distance runner. The first value, the lowest, is the 'acceleration speed'. The other two values are often very similar: the faster is the 'maximal speed'. Both the acceleration speed and maximal speed are higher in the sprinter. As in the subjects considered in **13.2**, in adolescents the acceleration phase is usually completed in the first 10m, and the maximal speed is usually reached between 20m and 30m.

Energy mechanisms evaluated by the test

The test is performed using almost exclusively the anaerobic mechanisms due to their rapid activation. Thus, subjects having high percentages of fast-twitch muscle fibres and in whom the anaerobic mechanisms are particularly well developed, obtain the best results. Among these subjects, those with more highly developed muscle masses have an additional advantage.

The Conconi test

In 1982 our research group developed a field test relating speed (S) to heart rate (HR) during incremental running.[3] Results show that the S–HR relationship is linear at low to moderate speeds and curvilinear at submaximal speeds. It is possible to identify the speed corresponding to the passage from the linear to the curvilinear phase, the so-called speed of deflection (S_d), which coincides with the anaerobic threshold (**13.3**). The routine application of this test has enabled us to refine the methodology of its execution and our results analysis.

Test procedure

Physical status of test subject

The test subject should be well rested and should not have performed hard physical work during the previous 48 hours. An intense workout, from which the subject has not yet recovered, modifies the S–HR relationship and may reduce the maximal HR, thus influencing the outcome of the test.

Warm-up

Our experience has shown that, in incremental tests of short duration (7–10min), a subject reaches his maximal HR only after a sufficient warm-up.

.3

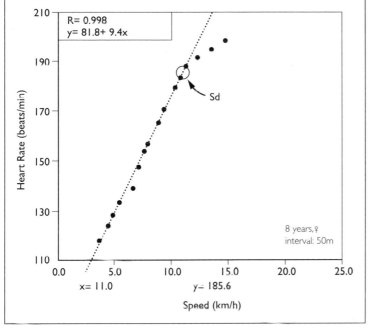

Warm-up time and intensity should be based upon the subject's age and physical conditioning (amount and intensity of regular physical activity). In general, the older and the more fit the subject, the longer the required warm-up time. Our warm-up protocol for children and untrained individuals consists of 10–15min of incremental physical activity of moderate intensity. Trained athletes perform a more vigorous incremental warm-up of at least 30min, with possible variations in work intensity.

Speed increase during the test: start-up to submaximal

In the past, we used protocols[3] that depended upon increasing speed after specific distances: we began with increments every 1000m (feasible only for long-distance runners), then we shortened the distance to 400m and 200m. Identical S–HR relationships were found, regardless of the distance used. It is well known that, with each increase in speed, the anaerobic mechanism comes into play (oxygen debt) until the aerobic metabolism adapts to the new work intensity. For this reason, the previous increments in speed after a given distance have been substituted, in the present protocol, by a gradual and practically continuous acceleration. Such acceleration must be not only gradual, but also small enough to minimize the employment of the anaerobic mechanism.

In practical terms, this requirement can be satisfied in the following way: after the warm-up, the subject begins the test at a work intensity that is low to moderate for his capabilities. The work output must be increased slightly and continuously, in such a way as to increase the corresponding HR by 8 beats per min or less, each minute. In addition, in order to obtain valid and consistent results, the test should last at least 7min, and preferably longer. Tests of shorter duration are usually accompanied by increases in HR greater than 8 beats per min each minute and lead to invalid results.

Speed increase during final part of the test

The slow constant increments of the initial part of the test must be substituted in the final part by fast incremental efforts up to the maximal speed. This final phase is begun when the subject being tested (or the test assistant) becomes aware of the physical signs of near-maximal effort, such as 'burning muscles' or breathing difficulties. These sensations of discomfort of the athlete at near maximal effort occur after the deflection point.

Pacing the athlete under test

There are several ways in which to control the subject's speed or work output and to guide his progression during the test up to submaximal speed: especially in children or in inexperienced subjects we prefer to 'pace' the subject with a bicycle equipped with a speedometer to control the subject's speed and to monitor his progression.

13.4

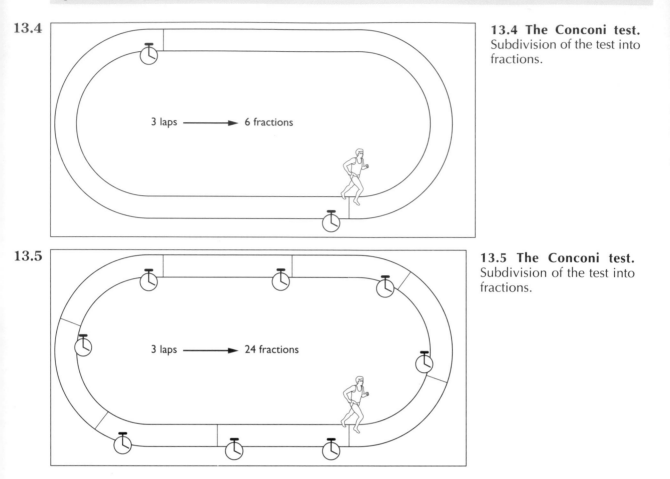

3 laps ⟶ 6 fractions

13.5

3 laps ⟶ 24 fractions

Subdivision of the test into fractions

One important aspect of the protocol is the subdivision of the test into fractions. The gradual continuous progression must be subdivided into as many intervals as necessary to collect sufficient data points to allow for good test analysis. For example, times could be taken every 200m (at the 200m and 400m marks of an athletic track). In this case, a test of 3 laps would be subdivided into 6 fractions (**13.4**). If times were taken every 100m, the same three-lap test would yield 12 data points. If, finally, times were taken every 50m, 24 data points would be obtained (**13.5**).

An example of the test carried out in a 9-year-old boy, and subdivided into intervals of different lengths, is shown in **13.6**. The graph has three out-of-phase ordinates to separate the three sets of data and allow for their comparison. When measurements are made every 200m, the straight line is well-defined, while the expected curvilinear section is not. In fact, only the last point is outside the straight line, which could be interpreted as an experimental error. When measurements are made every 100m, three points fall outside the straight

line. The curvilinear section is even more well-defined when measurements are taken every 50m. Therefore, measurements made every 50m seem to give the best results, especially when evaluating children.

Data measurement and analysis

During the test, HR and S are measured. We monitor HR continuously using a heart rate monitor with memory (Sport Tester PE 3000, Polar Electro, Kempele, Finland). The average HR for each interval can be calculated from the memorised data. The average S for each interval is calculated from elapsed time, measured with a stopwatch, photocells, or the Sport Tester itself. We have developed a computer program that allows automatic data transfer from the memory of the heart rate monitor to a computer and subsequent data analysis.

The analysis is carried out as follows:

- Following data transfer, the computer program calculates, for every test section, the average speed and the corresponding average heart rate. The scales of the graph are adjusted to the values of the collected data.

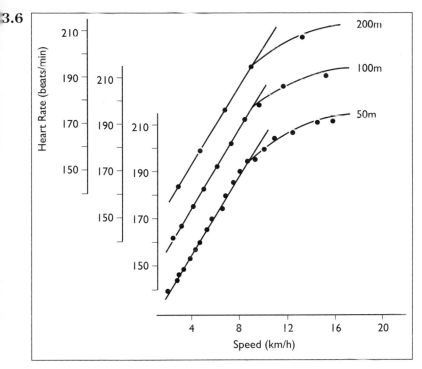

13.6 The Conconi test. Subdivision of the test into fractions.

• The program calculates the equations of all possible straight lines passing through the data points, as well as the corresponding correlation coefficients (r). The deflection point is identified as the point at which the values of the slope of the linear section and of the correlation coefficient begin to decrease. In a good test, these mathematical calculations are not necessary; the straight line can be traced manually and the deflection point can be easily identified subjectively with no significant errors.

Reproducibility of test results

The reproducibility of the S-HR relationship has been examined in several children and adolescents. A comparison of the results of two tests for a subject in running is presented in **13.7**. Almost identical straight-line equations and speed and heart rate at deflection were obtained. Any variations should occur only in the curvilinear portion of the test, that is, where the subjective motivation to obtain the highest possible speed comes into play. The subjective element does not interfere with the linear part of the test. Analysis of numerous tests indicates that, when the test is repeated within a few days and under constant experimental conditions, superimposable S-HR relationships are obtained.

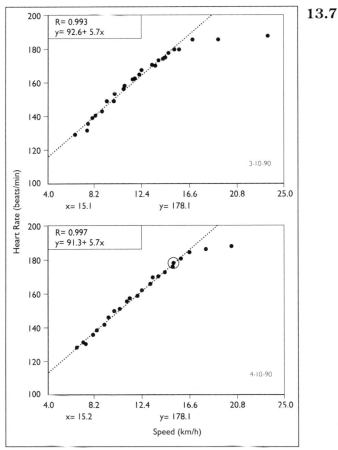

13.7

13.7 The Conconi test. Comparison of results between two tests.

13.8

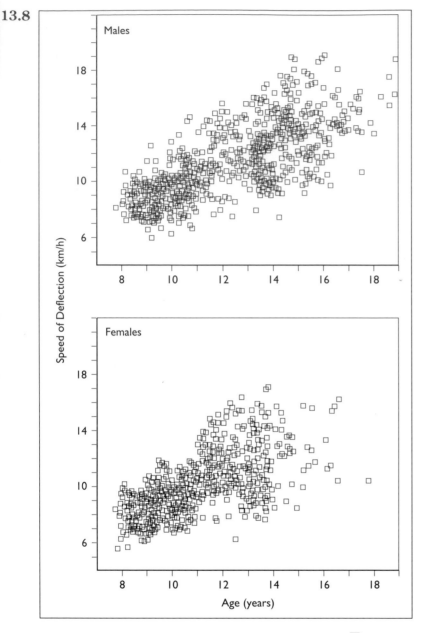

Modification of speed of deflection with age and training

Speed of deflection rises gradually with increasing age in both males and females (**13.8**). The values obtained among pre-pubertal subjects are rather closely grouped, while those for post-pubertal subjects are more dispersed, a phenomenon linked both to developmental differences during puberty and to variations in amount and type of physical activity. In particular, aerobic exercise is followed by increases in speed of deflection. These increases vary from subject to subject, indicating that both training and genetic factors influence these results.[1]

Energy mechanisms evaluated by the test

The speed of deflection values express the power (but not the endurance) of the aerobic metabolism, giving indications on 'how fast' (but not 'how long') one can go while using the aerobic mechanism.

Test to measure anaerobic power

A test to evaluate anaerobic lactacid power was developed in runners.[2] The test requires the determination of the average speed reached in an

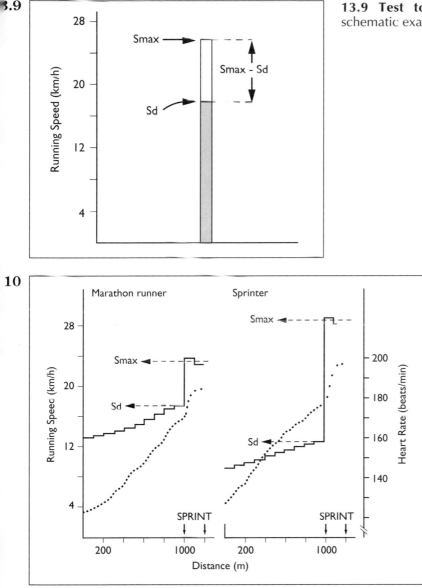

13.9 Test to measure anaerobic power. A schematic example.

13.10 Test to measure anaerobic power. Average speeds and the corresponding HR obtained during the test by a marathon runner and a sprinter.

all-out 200m sprint starting from a speed corresponding to the anaerobic threshold.

Test procedure

This test is carried out after determining the speed of deflection of the subject by means of the Conconi test. The subject to be tested is instructed to reach his speed of deflection progressively over 1000m and then to run another 200m at his highest possible speed. The final 200m is timed, and the corresponding speed calculated (maximal speed, S_{max}). The speed exceeding speed of deflection, calculated by subtracting S_d from S_{max}, is called

anaerobic speed (S_{an}). A schematic example is given in **13.9**.

This test has been adapted for children and adolescents by reducing the distance to reach S_d to 800m, and the all-out sprint to 100m.

Results

The average speeds and the corresponding HR obtained during the test by a marathon runner and a sprinter are shown in **13.10**. For purposes of data analysis, these two tests were subdivided into twelve 100m fractions. The anaerobic speed was much greater in the sprinter.

13.11

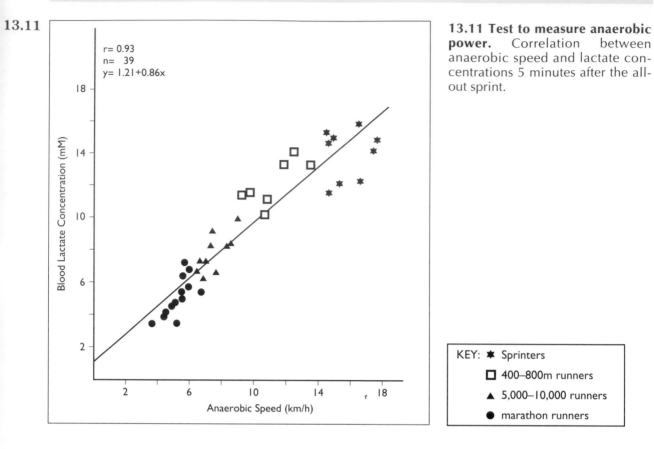

r= 0.93
n= 39
y= 1.21+0.86x

Blood Lactate Concentration (mM)

Anaerobic Speed (km/h)

13.11 Test to measure anaerobic power. Correlation between anaerobic speed and lactate concentrations 5 minutes after the all-out sprint.

KEY: ✱ Sprinters
□ 400–800m runners
▲ 5,000–10,000 runners
● marathon runners

Speeds generated above S_d are obtained primarily through the activation of the anaerobic lactacid metabolism, as shown by the correlation between anaerobic speed and lactate concentrations determined 5min after the all-out sprint (**13.11**). Both the anaerobic speeds and the lactate concentrations of the athletes considered in this study were in keeping with their characteristics, being highest for sprinters and decreasing progressively to 400–800m runners, to 5,000–10,000m runners, and to marathon runners. (Logically, also S_d, a measure of aerobic power, was significantly higher for the marathon and middle-distance runners than for the sprinters.)

Energy mechanisms evaluated by the test

This test measures the speed generated in runners by anaerobic glycolysis and excludes the speed generated by aerobic glucose breakdown. It overcomes the problems inherent in standing-start tests, namely:

- Progressive activation of the aerobic mechanism of ATP resynthesis.
- Individual variations in relative power and possibly in activation time of the various mechanisms of energy production.

- The contribution of creatine phosphate, which is negligible under the present test conditions.

Therefore, this test can be used to determine the power output generated by the lactacid anaerobic mechanism in various individuals and the effects of various training protocols on anaerobic glycolysis. The anaerobic speed expresses the power and not the endurance of anaerobic glycolysis, giving indications of 'how fast' but not 'how long' one can go while using this energy production modality.

The Cooper test

In 1968 Cooper described a field test for the evaluation of aerobic power. The Cooper test is a simulated race and consists of determining the distance covered in 12min of running.[4] In young active individuals, that distance is correlated to maximal oxygen consumption. However, in this maximal test, the anaerobic lactacid mechanism is utilised in addition to the aerobic mechanism. We wish to relate here our experience regarding the evaluation of the contribution of these two energy mechanisms, rendered possible by the joint application of the Cooper and Conconi tests.

12

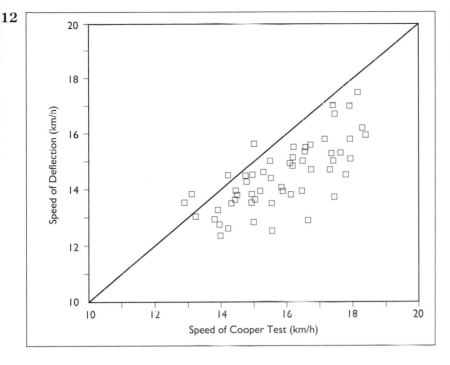

Joint application of the Cooper and Conconi tests

The Cooper test was conducted on a group of trained adolescents upon whom the Conconi test had been previously performed, with determination of speed of deflection. The Cooper test was carried out on a 400m track. During the test, the speed for each lap and the corresponding heart rate were determined.

13.12 presents the correlation between the average speed maintained during the Cooper test and S_d. Of the 60 adolescents tested, 56 ran at average speeds that exceeded their S_d, which confirms employment of the anaerobic lactacid mechanism during the Cooper test.

Further confirmation can be found in the data reported in **13.13**, which presents the lap speeds during the Cooper test for six of the subjects. The horizontal line represents the S_d, previously determined by means of the Conconi test:

- Subjects 2, 3 and 6 maintained speeds higher than S_d for the duration of the Cooper test.
- Subject 5 exceeded S_d in the initial and final phases.
- Subjects 1 and 4 ran faster than S_d only at the beginning of the test.

These different behaviours are representative of all of the subjects examined on this and other occasions.

Additional information can be obtained by continuous heart rate monitoring during the Cooper test. The heart rate values corresponding to the speed of deflection are always surpassed by the subjects, a further indication of the employment of the anaerobic lactacid mechanism during the Cooper test. However, the heart rates at the deflection are not attained immediately during the Cooper test but at different times in different subjects. This suggests that the cardiocirculatory adaptation to the effort varies from subject to subject as does the accumulation of an oxygen debt.

Energy mechanisms evaluated by the Cooper test

The test represents an important synthesis between the power of the aerobic mechanism and the power and capacity of the anaerobic lactacid mechanism. The joint application of the Cooper and Conconi tests allows information on aerobic power and on the differences in individual capacity to utilise the anaerobic lactacid mechanism in the Cooper test to be obtained.

Acknowledgement

This work was supported by Scuola dello Sport, Italian Olympic Committee, Rome.

13.13

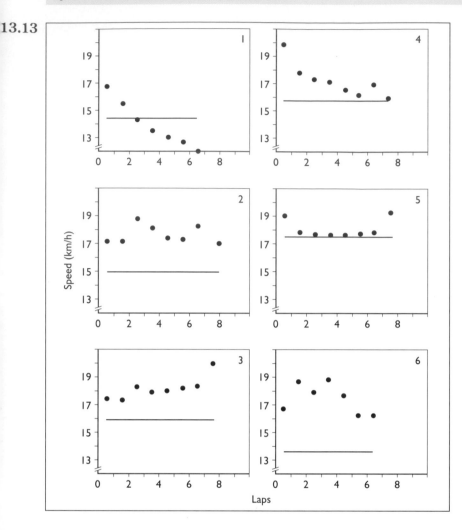

13.13 The Cooper test. Lap speeds during the Cooper test for six of the athletes in **13.12**.

References

1. Ballarin, E., Borsetto, C., Cellini, M., Patracchini, M., Vitiello, P., Ziglio, P.G. and Conconi, F. (1989) Adaptation of the 'Conconi test' to children and adolescents. *Int. J. Sports Med.* **10**: 334–338.
2. Borsetto, C., Ballarin, E., Casoni, I., Cellini, M., Vitiello, P. and Conconi, F. (1989) A field test for determining the speed obtained through anaerobic glycolysis in runners. *Int. J. Sports Med.* **10**: 339–345.
3. Conconi, F., Ferrari, M., Ziglio, P.G., Droghetti, P. and Codeca, L. (1982) Determination of the anaerobic threshold by a non-invasive field test in runners. *J. Appl. Physiol.: Resp. Env. Exerc. Physiol.* **52**: 869–873.
4. Cooper, K.H.A. (1968) A means of assessing maximal oxygen intake. *J. Amer. Med. Assoc.* **203**: 135–138.
5. Committee of Experts on Sports Research, Council of Europe. (1988) In: CONI, documentation and information division (Eds), Handbook for the Eurofit Tests of Physical Fitness, Rome.

Suggested reading

Maffulli, N., Capasso, G. and Lancia, A. (1991) Anaerobic threshold and performance in middle and long distance running. *J. Sports Med. Phys. Fit.* **31**: 332–338.

Maffulli, N., Greco, R., Greco, L. and D'Alterio, D. (1994) Treadmill exercise in Neapolitan children and adolescents. *Acta Paediatr.* **83**: 106–112.

Maffulli, N., Sjodin, B. and Ekblom, B. (1987) A laboratory method for non invasive anaerobic threshold determination. *J. Sports Med. Phys. Fit.* **27**: 419–423.

Maffulli, N. and Testa, V. (1991) Competitive marathon training. *J. Human Mov. Studies* **20**: 229–237.

Maffulli, N., Testa, V., Lancia, A., Capasso, G. and Lombardi, S. (1991) Indices of sustained aerobic power in young middle distance runners. *Med. Sci. Sports Exer.* **23**: 1090–1096.

14. The Role of Accident and Emergency in Paediatric Sports Emergencies

Manolis Gavalas, John Myers and Nicola Maffulli

Introduction

Sport is not just an important part of everyday life, enhancing good mental and physical health but also, to an increasing number of talented youngsters, it has become the passport to wealth and unique achievement.

Unfortunately, and in the United Kingdom in particular, facilities for the treatment of sports injuries not only do not exist but the injuries have been labelled as 'self inflicted'.

Accident and Emergency (A&E), in itself a new speciality which in theory should be dealing with all emergencies in addition to life- or limb-threatening situations, is in practice the reluctant and often the only protagonist for many sports injuries, offering regrettably suboptimal care.

Life-threatening emergencies

Deaths or critical conditions are mainly due to injuries associated with high-risk sports such as horse riding, car racing, karate and hang gliding. Accidents associated with swimming, scuba, Olympic diving and water-skiing have unchanging casualty numbers of drowning.

Trauma seen in team sports such as American football, soccer and rugby is a consequence of these sports' increasing popularity and participation by children at all competitive levels. Sport in which body contact is the accepted 'norm', and games with velocity objects, are high on the list causing death, due to head and neck injuries and cardiac contusion. Penetrating neck, chest or abdominal injuries seen in fencing, are rare but potentially very serious.

Non-traumatic deaths are essentially due to undiagnosed cardiac conditions. Fatalities due to exercise-induced asthma or diabetes are very uncommon. Thermo-regulatory impairment fatalities should be preventable, although heat stroke and hypothermia still cause death.

Optimum pre-hospital care with rapid triage and safe transport to emergency departments is matched by adherence to and practice of advanced trauma and cardiac life-support doctrines and protocols.

Trauma

The crucial role of A&E is to provide a fully-equipped resuscitation area, staffed with senior doctors proficient in paediatric resuscitation. The golden rule of managing any injured child is the uninterrupted perfusion of vital organs. A positive response from the child to the question: 'What is your name?' indicates an open airway, intact ventilation and adequate circulation and perfusion. At the same time, the team leader receives vital information from pre-hospital personnel.

A rapid **primary evaluation** and simultaneous treatment of life-threatening emergencies regardless of the type of injury always takes priority.

Airway maintenance with cervical spine control

In the spontaneously-breathing injured child, establishing a patent airway and administering supplemental oxygen is achieved by clearing the oropharynx and using the chin lift or jaw thrust manoeuvre, avoiding any neck movement. If there is any suspicion of a cervical spine injury the neck should be immobilised at all times, either manually or using a hard collar, sand bags and a tape.

Altered sensorium, agitation or subtle sounds may indicate a critically compromised airway. The pulse oximeter is a vital monitoring adjunct not a substitute for careful clinical assessment.

Failure of the above measures to maintain the airway after insertion of a correct size oropharyngeal airway necessitates orotracheal intubation with

14.1

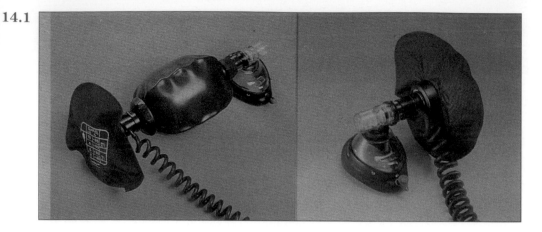

14.1 Assisted ventilation with 100% oxygen and maximum inspiratory supplemental oxygen concentration for the spontaneously breathing child can be achieved using standard resuscitation equipment. Demonstrated is the AmbuMark III ® resuscitator. (Reproduced courtesy of Ambu ® International (UK).)

in-line manual neck immobilisation to protect the 'injured until proven otherwise' cervical spine and correct application of Sellick's manoeuvre to lessen the risk of aspiration.

Inability to intubate the trachea demands a surgical airway. This is simple to perform and can be life-saving. For a child under 12 years of age, 12–14G cannula needle cricothyroidotomy and jet ventilation with oxygen at 40–50psi is preferred to surgical cricothyroidotomy, which is reserved for the older child.

Breathing and ventilation

Airway patency does not mean adequate ventilation. A Tension Pneumothorax is never a radiological diagnosis. It is identified by tracheal deviation, respiratory distress and a unilateral silent chest. Pulse oximetry shows a warning rapid desaturation and tachycardia. This grave emergency needs immediate needle decompression followed by insertion of a chest drain.

Until the patient is stable, oxygenation is achieved using a mask with a reservior bag device or mechanical ventilation using a mask-valve-bag device or a standard anaesthetic circuit (Bain), ensuring maximum FIO_2 or 100% oxygen, respectively.

A respiratory rate over $20.min^{-1}$ in the adolescent or $30.min^{-1}$ in the younger child indicates possible respiratory distress.

Circulation

In contrast to the adult, recognition of evolving shock can be extremely difficult to detect. Carotid pulse, heart rate, level of consciousness and skin circulation should be carefully assessed, bearing in mind that the increased physiologic reserve of the fit young athlete can mask vital signs. The normal blood volume in a child is in excess of $80\ ml.kg^{-1}$ Loss of 25% blood volume manifests with normotension, tachycardia (over $120.min^{-1}$ in the adolescent and over $140.min^{-1}$ in the younger child), altered level of consciousness and impaired capillary return and urinary output.

Frank systolic hypotension [normal systolic blood pressure in mmHg (B.P.) = 80 + (2 × age)] indicates a decompensated circulatory state with brady/tachydysrhythmias on the cardiac monitor, unrousability, pallor, cold skin and minimal urine output. At least 40% of blood volume has been lost and the child is minutes away from death or organ hypoxic damage.

Resuscitation starts immediately by administering high FIO_2 oxygen therapy, ensuring venous access and sending blood for cross-matching and baseline investigations. Pressure is applied to obvious external bleeding points and 20–40ml.kg^{-1} of warm crystalloid infusion is administered via two wide-bored cannulae. Poor response requires type O-RH-negative blood (10ml.kg^{-1}) or alternatively type-specific blood (20ml.kg^{-1}) if available, whilst urgent surgical intervention is arranged. Insertion of a nasogastric tube and urinary catheter is desirable unless contraindicated

If venous access proves impossible, alternatives include direct cut down or the intraosseous approach for the younger child.

Circulatory compromise in the young athlete is most often seen following abdominal and pelvic injuries in horse-riding accidents or falls.

Disability of neurological status

The child's level of consciousness is rapidly estimated using the A.V.P.U. method (A: Alert; V: Vocally-induced response; P: Pain-induced response; U: Unresponsive) and the size, symmetry and reactions of pupils to light are noted.

Exposure of the child

The child should be undressed completely taking care to avoid excessive heat loss. Cardiorespiratory stabilisation is followed by radiographs of the cervical spine, chest and pelvis in the Resuscitation Bay. Even if the lateral cervical spine X-ray shows all seven vertebrae and the C7/T1 junction to be normal, if the mechanism is suggesting neck trauma, movement of the neck should be prevented until a specialist excludes any cervical spine injury.

A **secondary evaluation** of the cardiovascularly-stable child is a total examination aiming to identify any evolving life-threatening injuries such as extradural haematoma, potential limb or career-threatening injuries, and detect and record all injuries irrespective of severity.

Head injuries

The majority of cases are minor and moderate, but severe head injuries cause fatalities and considerable morbidity. Following exclusion of an extracranial injury, the role of the A&E Department is to determine which child needs immediate neurosurgical intervention, which patient needs admission for observations and who can be safely discharged home.

The minor head injuries, with normal neurology and no initial loss of consciousness, can be safely allowed home with clear, written and understood head-injury instructions. Unless guidelines are nationally and internationally drawn and agreed, indications for skull X-rays will remain controversial. Some clear indications include clinical suspicion of a penetrating or depressed fracture.

In the more severe cases, a management protocol is followed in which a child with a G.C.S.≤8 or a deterioration of 2–3 points with or without a lateralised motor deficit and/or unequal pupils should be urgently intubated, hyperventilated, and CT scanned enroute to a neurosurgical facility for an evacuation of a probable haematoma.

In the comatose patient, absence of motor deficit or pupillary asymmetry suggests Diffuse Axonal Injury (DAI), which requires CT scan and intensive care neuromonitoring, bearing in mind that children develop raised Intracranial Pressure without focal mass lesions.

Absence of coma (G.C.S.>8) but with lateralised motor deficit indicates an expanding lesion and again requires CT scanning and neurosurgical referral.

History of prolonged loss of consciousness or post-traumatic amnesia or any abnormal neurology requires admission and early CT scanning.

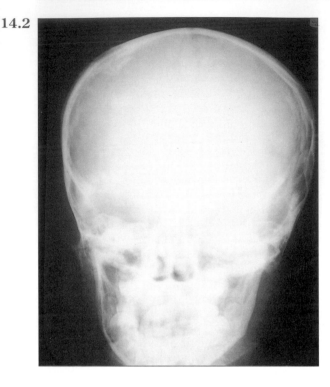

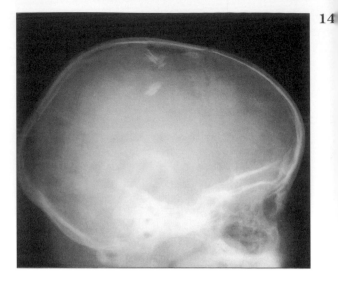

14.2, 14.3 Radiograph shows a comminuted depressed right parietal fracture with overlying soft tissue swelling and a bone fragment in the wound of an 11-year-old male amateur horse rider. He had fallen and sustained a serious head injury.

Skull fractures

Although diagnosing a skull fracture is important, brain injury does not depend on it. Obtaining a skull radiograph in some instances will only result in wasting precious time. Nevertheless, the presence of a fracture does identify the child with a higher probability of intracranial complications. Radiography may also show fluid levels, indicating paranasal involvement, or air in the cranium, but basal fractures are essentially diagnosed clinically (haemotympanum, CSF leaks, mastoid and peri-orbital ecchymosis).

Post-concussion syndrome

It is common in its mild form and presents with vertigo, headaches, nausea and dizziness. There is no positive neurology and in the majority of cases, responds to simple analgesia and rest.

Scalp wounds

These can cause troublesome bleeding in children, but usually heal well if general principles of wound management are followed. Prior to suture, it is vital to palpate the wound for depressed fractures.

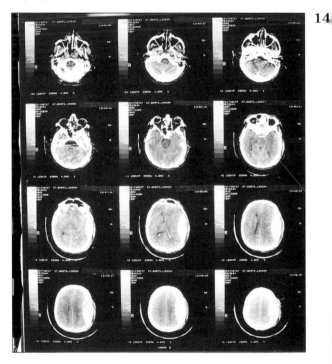

14.4 The CT scan after exclusion of extracranial injuries shows a right extradural haematoma, ipsilateral compression of the ventricular anatomy, obliteration of the sylvian fissure, mass effect and a small quantity of air in the cranium of a 16-year-old amateur climber who fell and sustained a head injury. He had a G.C.S. of 8 and lateralised deficit.

14.5 Radiograph shows a right parietal fracture in an 8-year-old girl who fell off her horse and lost consciousness.

14.5

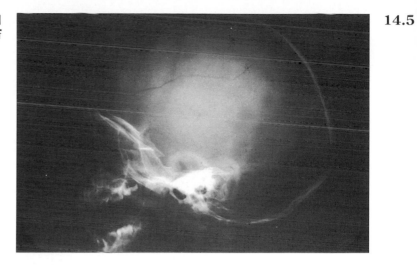

.6

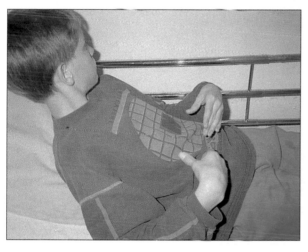

14.6 Classical carpopedal spasm, due to hyperventilation in a 13-year-old boy who was involved in an accidental clash of heads during a football match. He was subdued, looking extremely distressed and tearful, and was subsequently taken to A&E. There was no neurological deficit.

14.7

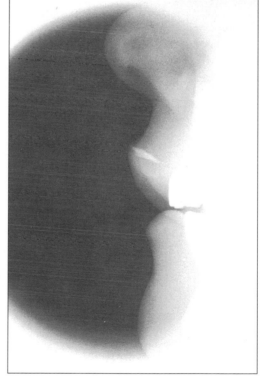

14.7 This radiograph illustrates a facial wound, containing a foreign body, sustained by a 14-year-old girl point-to-point horse rider after a fall. Such foreign bodies must always be excluded from all wounds.

14.8

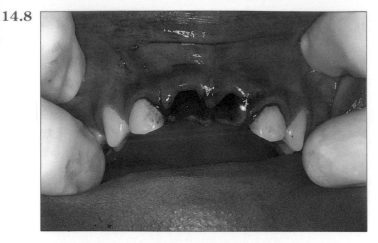

14.8 An illegal blow received by a 14-year-old male martial arts amateur from the foot of his opponent avulsed both of his incisors. (Reproduced courtesy of Jane Goodman, Consultant in Paediatric Dentistry, Eastman Dental Hospital.)

14.9

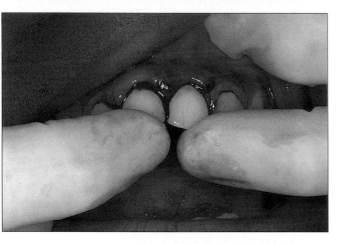

14.9 Successful reimplantation in A&E and subsequent referral to a paediatric dentist. (Reproduced courtesy of Jane Goodman, Consultant in Paediatric Dentistry, Eastman Dental Hospital.)

14.10

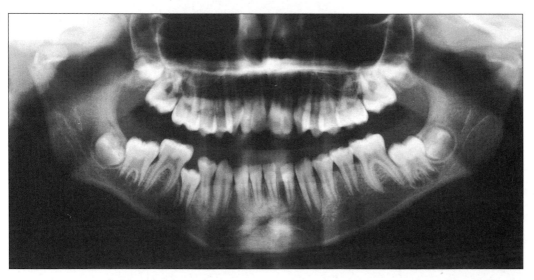

14.10 The radiograph shows bilateral fractures of the mandibular condyles of a 16-year-old rugby player, indicating a considerable force impact on the lower jaw. He was tackled heavily by two opponents falling on his face from a height, whilst attempting a spectacular dive.

Maxillo-facial trauma

Fractures of the nasal bones seen in older children can cause considerable soft-tissue swelling. Radiography in the young is unnecessary as there is no bony skeleton. Non-urgent early referral to an ENT specialist is indicated, provided a septal haematoma is excluded. This is common in children as the mucoperichondrium is loosely attached to the cartilage. The bulging mass on inspection is characteristic. If left undetected, it may cause cartilage necrosis, abscess formation and subsequently collapse of the nose or, rarely, cavernous sinus thrombosis.

'Blow out' fractures of the orbit seen typically with squash-ball injuries cause extensive haematoma of the eyelid. Ruptures of the orbital wall cause enophthalmos and diplopia. Radiology may show the teardrop sign.

Isolated zygomatic-arch fracture is common but recognition of a tripod fracture is difficult because of soft-tissue swelling. Infra-orbital steps or sensory impairment may be the only signs present.

Antibiotic cover for unrecognised CSF leaks and involvement of a specialist is essential practice.

Laryngotracheal trauma

Although very uncommon in sports injuries, it can occur with racquet sports or blows to the neck in tae kwon do, karate or basketball. Classically, the hyoid bone fractures causing severe pain on swallowing or palpation. Surgical emphysema indicates breaking of the laryngeal lumen. These injuries need urgent specialist referrals.

Auricular trauma

Auricular haematoma should be treated under strict aseptic conditions by aspiration, bandage pressure and specialist follow-up, as further treatment may be necessary.

Lacerations of the auricle need specialist plastic-surgery referral if extensive or if cartilage is left exposed. Simple lacerations need suturing and antibiotic cover.

Eye injuries

Ten percent of all sports-related eye injuries occur in racquet sport. Ice hockey still causes 'a few too many' blind eyes. It is mandatory to measure and

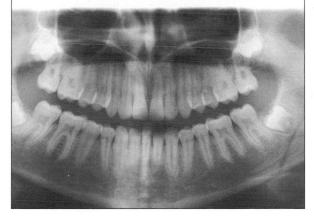

14.11

14.11 Radiograph shows fracture of left ramus of 16-year-old male Afro-Caribbean boxer, a very unusual boxing injury.

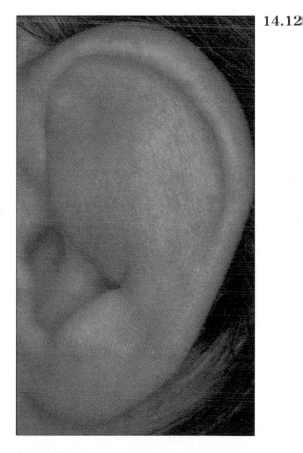

14.12

14.12 Blunt trauma to the pinna may cause a seroma. This must be treated with respect and always referred to the ENT specialist. (Reproduced with kind permission of Churchill Livingstone: *Clinical Otoscopy: A Text and Colour Atlas*.)

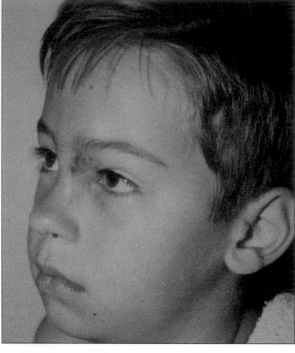

14

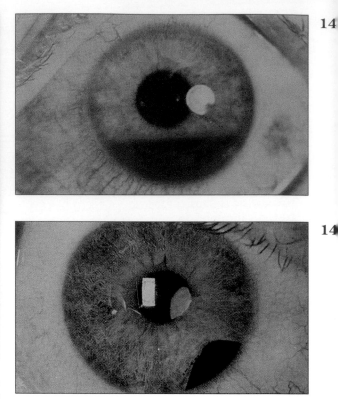

14

14.13 A hockey-stick injury to a 12-year-old boy, obtained during a school P.E lesson. In addition to racquet sports, orbital injuries can occur in lacrosse, ice hockey and hurling.

14.14, 14.15 Severe blows to the eye (racquet sports, ice hockey) can manifest with haemorrhage into the anterior chamber (hyphaema) and iris disinsertion (iridodialysis). (Reproduced with kind permission of Churchill Livingstone: *Clinical Opthalmology: A Text and Colour Atlas.*)

14.16

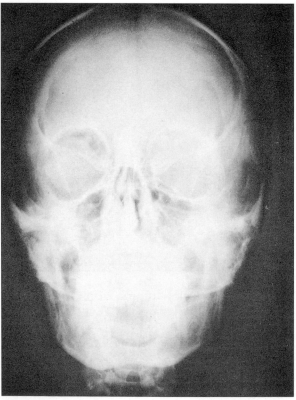

14.16 The presence of air in the orbit indicates a fracture necessitating urgent ophthalmological referral for a 15-year-old girl with a lacrosse injury to her right eye.

record the visual acuity in all injuries. Examining the anterior segment can be difficult due to blepharospasm. This can be overcome by the use of a topical anaesthetic. Retraction of the eyelids and visualisation of all the corneal surface is essential. Breaks in the cornea are seen with the aid of fluorescein stain under a U/V light. Traumatic mydriasis is common following blunt injury to the iris sphincter. Bleeding into the anterior segment causes hyphaema. Violent trauma can cause iridodialysis or retinal detachment. Except for minor trauma, all eye injuries need urgent specialist referral.

Spinal injuries

Although uncommon in children, these can account for up to 20% of all injuries seen in spinal units. In children aged 10–14 years, sport (recreational or organised) claims equal numbers of spinal injuries as road traffic trauma.

Diving into shallow water is a summertime epidemic accounting for 50% of all trauma, mostly cervical spine injuries. Risky sports include gliding, rugby, motor-cross, stock-car racing, sledging and ice hockey.

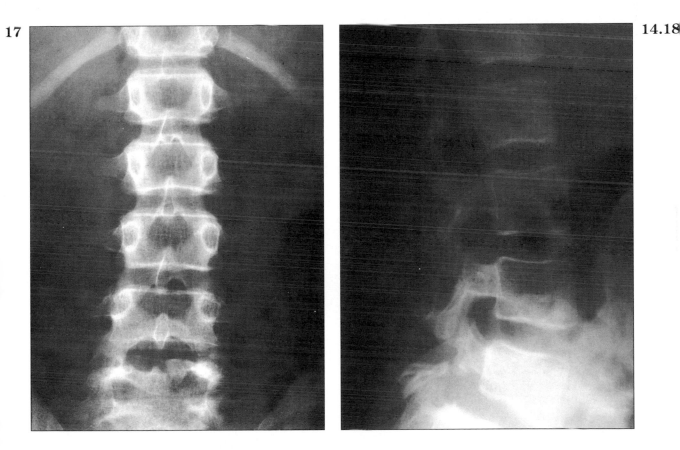

14.17, 14.18 X-ray shows bilateral pars interarticularis defects of L5 with grade one spondylolisthesis in an 11-year-old female gymnast who presented to A&E with severe backache following strenuous training. On examination, she had restricted flexion of her spine and impaired SLR. Backache in children is unusual and must be taken seriously, especially in sports such as weight lifting, ballet dancing, high jumping (Fosbury flop), butterfly swimming, rowing and rugby.

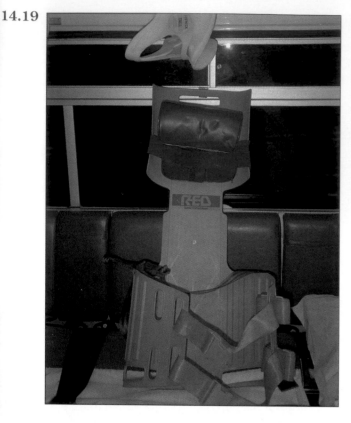

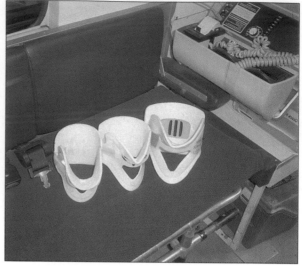

14.20 Various sizes of collars used in neck injuries. The A&E personnel should never rely entirely on any cervical collar by itself to guarantee immobilisation.

14.19 Equipment for spinal immobilisation by pre-hospital personnel.

Chest trauma

Cardiac contusion does occur in sport and is often missed in the emergency department. It is probably the most common unsuspected visceral injury responsible for death in a young athlete.

The principal clinical manifestation is ventricular dysrhythmia, the nature of which is unrelated to the size of contusion or the extent of morphological damage. It is important to treat these injuries with respect by continuous monitoring in the resuscitation area.

A twelve-lead ECG may show PVC's, non-specific ST and T wave changes and conduction impairment. Admission to an intensive care unit is essential, as sudden death from complete heart block is possible.

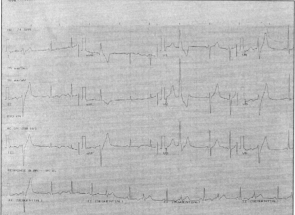

14.21 This ECG shows multifocal PVCs and bigemini in a 16-year-old male cricketer accidentally struck on chest by a cricket ball. He was brought to A&E complaining of giddiness and palpitations, and was admitted to ITU with suspected cardiac contusion.

Abdominal and genitourinary trauma

The possibility that an abdominal viscus is injured must always be considered. The innocent 'kick in the stomach' of the young goal-keeper could be hiding a splenic rupture. If in doubt, and provided that the child is haemodynamically normal and is

14.22 Radiograph of the pelvis of a 16-year-old boy shows an undisplaced fracture of his acetabulum. Whilst snow boarding abroad on holiday, he lost his balance in mid-air, and fell awkwardly on his left leg. He could not bear weight and apparently, radiographs of his left leg were normal. On returning to the UK, he presented to A&E in pain, limping and with a very restricted range of movement of his left hip. (Reproduced courtesy of the Accident and Emergency Department, St Bartholomew's Hospital, London.)

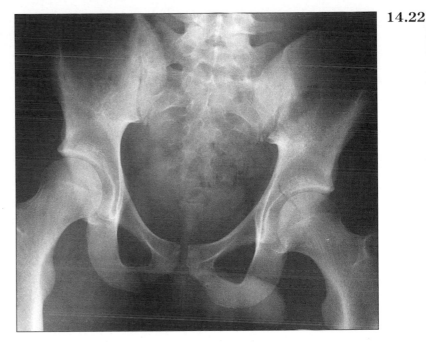

constantly monitored, urgent computed scanning should be arranged. Blood must always be sent for cross-matching and the urine tested for blood. No hesitancy should be shown in involving a paediatric surgeon.

Microscopic or macroscopic haematuria must be investigated with urgent I.V.P.

Blood in the urethral meatus or scrotal haematoma could indicate tears in the anterior urethra. Classically, these are seen in straddle sports injuries and contraindicate insertion of a urinary catheter.

Musculoskeletal injuries

Clinical examination methodically undertaken using inspection, palpation and movement is directed to the skin, vascular status of the limb, its nerve supply and to the possibility of damage to muscles or tendons, the bone itself or associated joint injury.

The possibility of infection following a sports **compound fracture,** particularly with sporulated micro-organisms such as clostridii, should always be borne in mind. The management of an open fracture is always the management of the wound with time being of the essence in preventing infection. In A&E, removal of gross contamination takes priority, assuming that vascular supply is unimpaired. The fracture should be aligned with proper splinting to control further damage and pain. Adequate parenteral analgesia must never be denied unless specifically contraindicated. The limb is X-rayed urgently and the wound is subsequently covered with sterile dressings often soaked in iodine solution. The use of instant photography enables the wound dressings to be left undisturbed. Antibiotic and tetanus prophylaxis are administered prior to specialist referral.

Fractures are very common in sport but fortunately complications are not. If present, they must not be missed. This can be achieved by remembering that if a bone is injured so can the associated structures. The skills of clinical examinations must never be allowed to give way to complacency.

Epiphyseal injuries should be managed by a paediatric orthopaedic specialist. Type V compression injuries are easy to miss in the emergency department. Considering an epiphyseal plate as injured until proven otherwise is a safe and wise policy.

In A&E iatrogenic **compartment syndrome** is always a possibility. Bivalving all casts and giving clear and easily understood written instructions for early recognition at home of this impending disaster is standard practice.

14.23

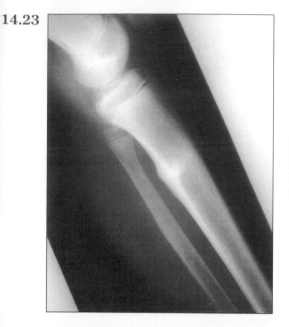

14.24

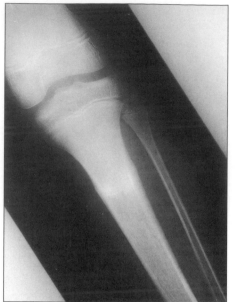

14.23, 14.24 X-rays show a healing stress fracture of the tibia with a clear periosteal reaction and focal sclerosis. A 15-year-old male jogging enthusiast presented with a history of pain in the left leg for four weeks, following a tackle he received in a football match.

14.25

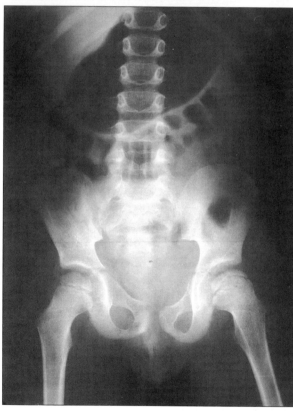

14

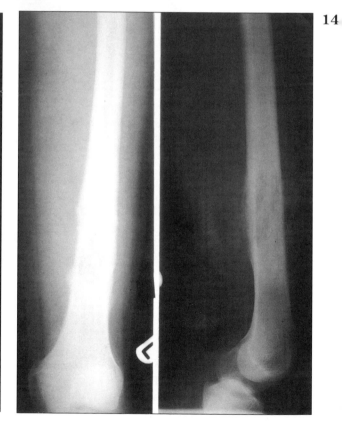

14.25 Pelvic X-ray of an 8-year-old boy involved in a motorbike scrambling accident. He was brought to A&E in hypovolaemic shock. The X-ray shows fractures of the superior and inferior pubic rami and iliac crest. Note coincidental left Perthes on the opposite side of the injury.

14.26 X-ray shows an osteogenic sarcoma diagnosed in a 16-year-old boy presented to A&E with a 10-day history of pain in his left thigh, following a rugby injury. Note the soft tissue mass representing a haematoma. It is not unusual for bone tumours to be diagnosed following coincidental trauma.

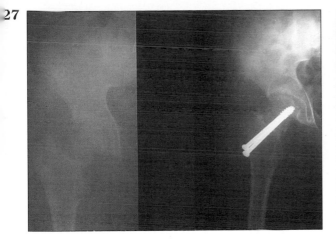

14.27 A fractured neck of femur was sustained by a 12-year-old girl whilst mountaineering. She was treated with cannulated screws.

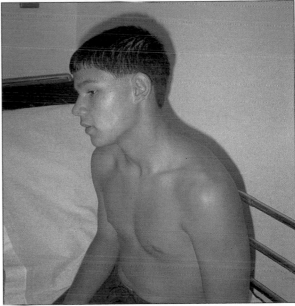

14.28 Acute torticollis is commonly seen in young athletes and is probably caused by minor soft tissue injury. It responds well to heat therapy, analgesia, soft collar support and rest.

Soft tissue injuries

The severity of a joint injury can be predicted by considering the mechanism of injury, whether the child was carried off and was unable to continue, the rapid joint swelling indicating a haemarthrosis, and the inability to bear weight on the injured limb.

Ankle sprain is a clinical diagnosis of exclusion, and X-rays are only indicated if there is doubt about the diagnosis or extent of trauma.

Muscle tears are common traumatic sports injuries in the adolescent. They can be slow to resolve but almost invariably respond to rest and physiotherapy.

All non-acute sports injuries and follow-ups of children seen in the emergency department with specific sports injuries should be the responsibility of a sports specialist. The management of the young athlete can be thus individualised for a most effective treatment and rehabilitation programme, ensuring a safe and quick return to physical activity.

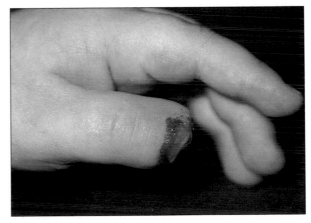

14.29 Three weeks post-traumatic appearance of the thumb of a 13-year-old boy, following an ice skating accident. These types of injury have an excellent prognosis provided that basic principles of wound management are followed.

Lacerations and wounds

Exclusion of associated neurovascular, bony and tendinous injury and of foreign bodies is essential management of these injuries. Exploration, irrigation, debridement and haemostasis under strict aseptic techniques and local anaesthesia is standard emergency practice. Leaving a dirty wound open for delayed primary suture is always wise. Tetanus prophylaxis with toxoid booster or Humotet according to current protocol must never be ignored.

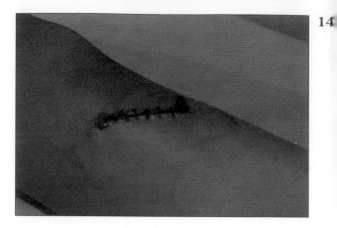

14.30 Laceration sustained by a 14-year-old boy during a marathon race. First aid consisted of inappropriate suturing of this potentially dirty wound. Subsequent presentation to A&E three days later with an obvious infection.

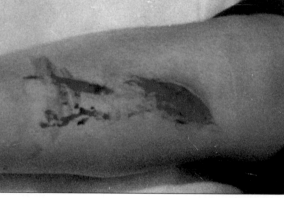

14.31 Stud wound injuries sustained by a 14-year-old male footballer, not wearing shin-guards, who was tackled illegally. The wound was cleaned and left open for delayed primary suture.

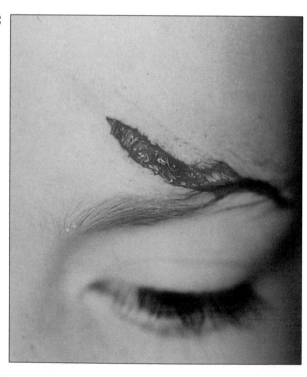

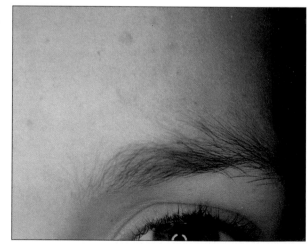

14.32, 14.33 A 12-year-old male footballer sustained this clean laceration following a head-to-head clash. The selective use of tissue adhesive (Histoacryl) offers good cosmetic results, avoids the use of local anaesthetic and is extremely time saving (Reproduced courtesy of Davis & Geck, B. Braun Melsungen).

Non-traumatic sports injuries

The vast majority of young athletes are healthy individuals with no previous history of cardio-vascular or other problems. Unfortunately, arrhythmias and other problems may suddenly become symptomatic and present to A&E either in full cardiorespiratory collapse, or with palpitations, dyspnoea, dizziness, syncope or bizarre neurological symptoms.

Exertional syncope in particular must never be taken lightly or labelled 'vasovagal', as it can be the only manifestation of malignant arrhythmias or congenital cardiac defect.

A history, which includes family history and establishes the timing of syncope in relation to the onset and severity of exertion, must always be taken. Chest pain associated with syncope with or without impaired tissue perfusion or premature ventricular contractions (PVCs) could be caused by an acute myocardial infarction or critical cardiac ischaemia.

Careful systematic examination, electrocardiography and beat-to-beat non-invasive monitoring of cardiac rhythm is standard emergency management of these children. ECG evidence of myocardial strain, conduction defects or ischaemia necessitates admission to coronary care.

Unless the hallmarks of syndromes (e.g. Marfans) associated with cardiac abnormalities are specifically sought for in the emergency room, young athletes will be denied early life-saving treatment and return to normal activities.

The role of the A&E specialist is not to offer precision of diagnosis [e.g. hypertrophic obstructive cardiomyopathy (HOCM) or right ventricular dysplasia], but to be suspicious that all is not normal and request urgent specialised evaluation by a cardiologist. Urgent investigations must always include a chest X-ray and one or more twelve-lead ECGs. The patient's vital signs should be continuously monitored with uninterrupted supervision during the entire duration of the child's care in the emergency department.

Arrhythmias such as Bigeminy, Trigeminy, R-on-T phenomena, Mobitz ll block, and multiple PVCs are always pathological. The ECG evidence of left ventricular hypertrophy is not necessarily indicative of athletic fitness.

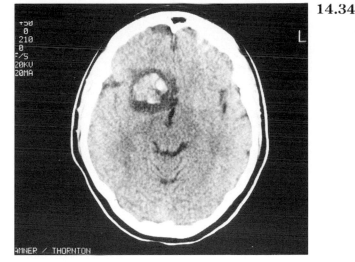

14.34

14.34 CT scan of a 13-year-old girl presented to A&E with headache, vomiting and photophobia, following strenuous physical activity at P.E. She had a similar but less severe episode the previous year, which resolved spontaneously. The scan shows a right frontal/temporal focal bleed surrounded by an oedematous halo with mild mass effect. This bleed was either coincidental or secondary to the presence of a vascular abnormality precipitated by high pressures exerted during strenuous exercise.

Cardiopulmonary resuscitation

With the exception of congenital heart abnormalities and hypovolaemia, hypoxia due to respiratory impairment almost invariably precedes cessation of spontaneous cardiac activity. This highlights the significance of pre-hospital basic life support. Advanced life support should always be based on current international guidelines.

Ventricular fibrillation and pulseless ventricular tachycardia respond well to defibrillation of initially 2 joules.kg^{-1}, but they are uncommon compared to asystole or EMD which carry a less favourable prognosis.

Regarding hypothermia, no child should be considered dead until core temperature registers normothermia.

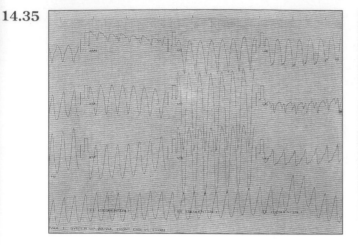

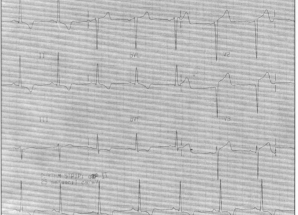

14.35 A 14-year-old boy presented with palpitations following strenuous activity during a swimming event. Whilst being assessed in A&E, his cardiovascular state deteriorated dramatically with his electrocardiogram showing ventricular tachycardia. He underwent emergency synchronised cardioversion and was admitted to ITU.

14.36 This ECG of a 16-year-old muscular rugby player, who presented to A&E with chest pain and dizziness following a collapse in a match, has enough tell-tale features of obstructive cardiomyopathy. Other ECG features of HOCM include Q waves in V5, V6, AVL and Lead I due to septal hypertrophy and decreased PR interval. The onset of AF is a very ominous sign.

Drowning and near-drowning

It is vitally important to restart the heart in the field as the majority of children who reach hospital with a cardiac output survive. A clear airway and high supplemental FIO_2 oxygen if the child is breathing spontaneously, or intubating and ventilating with 100% oxygen if the child is apnoeic, always takes priority. Chest compressions commence only if there is no output.

VF due to hypothermia is resistant to cardioversion until the core temperature rises. This also resolves other bradyarrhythmias. Initial non-invasive monitoring, estimation of arterial blood gases, chest X-ray, plasma expansion, antibiotics and correction of electrolyte and acid-base deficits is mandatory prior to admission to intensive care.

Exercise-induced asthma

Any sport, with the possible exception of swimming, can precipitate bronchoconstriction in an asthmatic young athlete. Severe attacks are managed with high FIO_2 therapy, nebulised bronchodilators (selective Beta$_2$ agonists and antimuscarinics) and steroids. Aminophylline or Salbutamol infusion is a second-line management reserved for those with a poor response, who must always be admitted. Subjective and objective response parameters dictate further management.

Diabetic complications

Public awareness of diabetes is growing and takes credit for the rare occurrence of hypoglycaemia amongst the young diabetic athletes of today. Both hypoglycaemia and hyperglycaemic ketotic attacks are managed with conventional emergency measures.

Heat stroke

The usual presentation is with severe hyperthermia, syncope, abnormal G.C.S., seizures and delirium. Abnormal vital signs are associated with severe cases. Emergency management is directed towards the airway and ventilation. Supplemental oxygen, volume expansion and slow cooling prior to admission to critical care is mandatory.

Hypothermia

Severe hypothermia (<30°C) secondary to immersion is not difficult to diagnose and requires critical care. Mild (32–35°C) and moderate (30–32°C) cases, seen following prolonged exposure in outdoor sports activities, can present subtly and may be missed unless special low-registering thermometers are used. In the A&E setting, monitoring of vital signs and passive external rewarming is required prior to admission.

14.37 The radiograph shows mediastinal emphysema in a 13-year-old male cross-country runner who presented to A&E with a moderate attack of asthma.

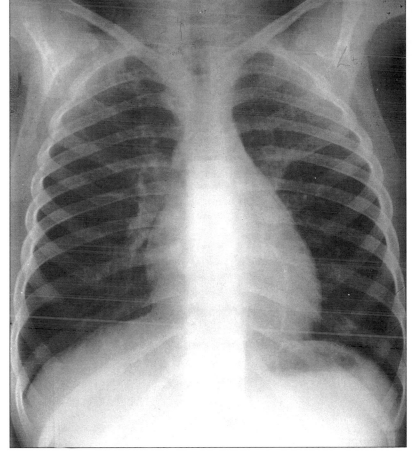

Scuba-diving accident

Drowning, air embolism, decompression sickness and accidental carbon monoxide poisoning are the commonest emergencies associated with this sport.

Air embolism due to to pulmonary barotrauma simulates a cerebrovascular accident. Often, visual impairment is a prominent feature. Pulmonary complications include mediastinal emphysema, pneumothorax and haemoptysis. The management of this emergency is support of the vital signs and hyperbaric decompression .

Decompression sickness can develop insidiously with a wide-ranging spectrum of signs. If spinal cord involvement is present, immediate recognition is vital ensuring supportive measures and rapid decompression to avoid permanent disability.

Accidental carbon monoxide poisoning can present acutely or insidiously, and can be difficult to diagnose if not suspected. Pulse oximetry is misleadingly normal, being unable to differentiate oxygen from carbon monoxide haemoglobin occupancy.

A&E treatment is essentially supportive with high-flow oxygen delivery for maximum FIO_2. Serious cases need urgent oxygenation in a recompression chamber.

Acknowledgement

With special thanks to Laura Cullum for her invaluable support.

14.38 Paediatric peak flow rate graph, available in A&E for assessing asthmatic children (Reproduced with kind permission of Clement Clarke International).

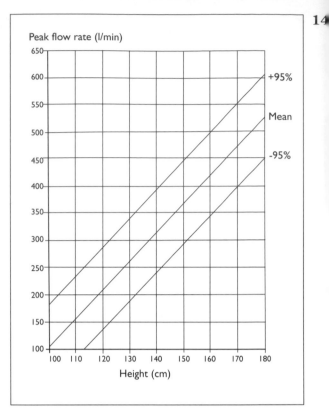

Suggested further reading

1. *Advanced Trauma Life Support Course* (1993) American College of Surgeons Student Manual.
2. Skinner, D.V. and Vincent, R. (1993) *Cardiopulmonary Resuscitation*, Chapter 9, Oxford University Press.
3. Avery, J.G., Harper, P. and Ackroyd, S. (1990) *Do We Pay Too Dearly For Our Sport and Leisure Activities?* Society of Public Health.
4. Mok, D.W.H. and Kreel, L. (1988) Essential radiology in head injury. In: *A Diagnostic Atlas of Skull Trauma*. BAS Printers Ltd, Oxford, UK.
5. Royal College of Physicians (1991) *Medical Aspects of Exercise: Benefits and Risks*, London.
6. Sports Council (1988) *Safety in Swimming Pools*. Sports Council, London.
7. McKenna, W.J. and Camm, A.J.C. (1989) Sudden death in hypertrophic cardiomyopathy – assessment of patients at high risk. *Circulation* **80**: 1489–1492.

Index